D0903239

Ethics in Health Education

Ethics in Health Education

Editor

SPYROS DOXIADIS
President, Foundation for Research in Childhood, Athens

Editorial Committee

Alastair V Campbell
Professor of Biomedical Ethics
Otago Medical School, Dunedin

R S Downie
Professor of Moral Philosophy
University of Glasgow, Glasgow

Lucien Karhausen
Research Fellow, Cortona

Susie Stewart
Technical Editor, Glasow

JOHN WILEY & SONS
Chichester · New York · Brisbane · Toronto · Singapore

Other Wiley Editorial Offices

John Wiley & Sons, Inc., 605 Third Avenue,
New York, NY 10158-0012, USA

Jacaranda Wiley Ltd, G.P.O. Box 859, Brisbane,
Queensland 4001, Australia

John Wiley & Sons (Canada) Ltd, 22 Worcester Road,
Rexdale, Ontario M9W 1L1, Canada

John Wiley & Sons (SEA) Pte Ltd, 37 Jalan Pemimpin #05-04,
Block B, Union Industrial Building, Singapore 2057

Library of Congress Cataloging-in-Publication Data:

Ethics in health education / editor, Spyros Doxiadis : editorial
   committee, Alastair Campbell . . . [*et al*.].
      p.   cm.
   Includes bibliographical references.
   ISBN 0 471 92606 X
   1. Health education—Moral and ethical aspects. I. Doxiadēs,
Spyros. II. Campbell, Alastair V.
R737.E84   1990
174'.2—dc20   89-28822
                                                      CIP

British Library Cataloguing in Publication Data:

Ethics in health education.
   1. Health education. Ethical aspects
   I. Doxiadis, Spyros
   174'.2

   ISBN 0 471 92606 X

Printed and bound by Biddles Ltd., Guildford, Surrey.

Contents

Acknowledgements vii

Contributors ix

Prologue xi
    Spyros Doxiadis

SECTION I   THEORETICAL BACKGROUND

1 Ethics in Health Education: An Introduction. 3
    R. S. Downie

2 Education or Indoctrination? The Issue of Autonomy in Health
   Education 15
    Alastair V. Campbell

3 Health Education: The Ambiguity of the Medical Role 29
    Raanan Gillon

SECTION II   SOCIOPOLITICAL ISSUES

4 Health Care Advertising: Communication or Confusion? 45
    Samuel Gorovitz

5 Health Education: The Political Tensions 63
    Stephen Pattison and David Player

6 The Role of Organized Medicine in the Ethics of Health Education
   and Health Promotion 81
    Ole K. Harlem

7 **The Journalist as Health Educator** 93
  Jean-Daniel Flaysakier

SECTION III   TARGET GROUPS

8 **Ethics of Health Education for Children** 107
  Spyros Doxiadis and Tina Garanis

9 **Health Education in Schools**. 125
  R. S. Downie and Carol Fyfe

10 **Health Education and Self-Care** 145
  Yannis C. Tountas

11 **Health Education and the AIDS Epidemic**. 155
  Leon Eisenberg

12 **Ethics, Health Education, and Nutrition**. 181
  Povl Riis

13 **Health Education and Mental Health** 191
  Jacqueline M. Atkinson

Epilogue. 209
  R. S. Downie

Index 211

Acknowledgements

I would like to thank the Commission of the European Communities for financial support. The Foundation for Research in Childhood in Athens has also contributed to the cost of this project and for this help I am extremely grateful. Thanks are also due to Tina Garanis for editorial help and to Anny Zahopoulou and Anna Frantzi for their administrative and secretarial assistance.

Without the expertise and commitment of our Technical Editor, Susie Stewart, the book would not have been published and I am greatly indebted to her.

Finally, I would like also to thank most warmly all the members of the Editorial Committee for their hard work and friendly cooperation, and all the authors for their willingness to contribute to the book and for all the work this involved.

SPYROS DOXIADIS
Athens, July 1989

Contributors

JACQUELINE M. ATKINSON *Lecturer, Department of Community Medicine, University of Glasgow, 2 Lilybank Gardens, Glasgow G12 8QQ, Scotland*

ALASTAIR V. CAMPBELL *Professor of Biomedical Ethics, Otago Medical School, P.O. Box 913, Dunedin, New Zealand*

R. S. DOWNIE *Professor of Moral Philosophy, Department of Philosophy, The University of Glasgow, Glasgow G12 8QQ, Scotland*

SPYROS DOXIADIS *Professor and President, Foundation for Research in Childhood, 42 Amalias Street, Athens 105 58, Greece*

LEON EISENBERG *Professor and Chairman, Department of Social Medicine and Health Policy, Harvard Medical School, 25 Shattuck Street, Boston, MA 02115, USA*

JEAN-DANIEL FLAYSAKIER *Chief Medical Editor, Antenne 2 – French Public TV, 22 Avenue Montaigne, 75387 Paris Cedex 08, France*

CAROL FYFE *Researcher, Department of Community Medicine, University of Glasgow, 2 Lilybank Gardens, Glasgow G12 8QQ, Scotland*

TINA GARANIS *Lawyer, Foundation for Research in Childhood, 42 Amalias Street, Athens 105 58, Greece*

RANAAN GILLON *Editor, Journal of Medical Ethics, c/o Imperial College Health Centre, 14 Prince's Gardens, London SW7 1NA, England*

SAMUEL GOROVITZ *Professor and Dean, College of Arts and Sciences, Syracuse University, 300 Hall of Languages, Syracuse, NY 13244-1170, USA*

OLE K. HARLEM *Paediatrician, Bruksvn 5, 1335 Snaroya, Norway*

LUCIEN KARHAUSEN *Research Fellow, c/o Ricci, S M Nuova 20, Cortona (Arezzo), Italy*

STEPHEN PATTISON *Secretary, Central Birmingham Community Health Council, 45 Bull Street, Birmingham B4 6AF, England*

DAVID PLAYER *District Medical Officer, South Birmingham Health Authority, Oak Tree Lane, Selly Oak, Birmingham B29 6JF, England*

POVL RIIS *Professor of Internal Medicine, University of Copenhagen, Herlev University Hospital, DK-2730 Herlev, Denmark*

SUSIE STEWART   *Technical Editor, 34 Rowan Road, Glasgow G41 5BZ, Scotland*
YANNIS C. TOUNTAS   *Assistant Professor of Social Medicine, Technological Institute of Athens, 7 P. Nirvana Street, Filothei 132 57, Athens, Greece*

Prologue

SPYROS DOXIADIS

While working with my co-authors for two previous books on aspects of medical ethics, of which I was the editor, we realized that there was an important part of ethics which had not been sufficiently described and discussed. This is the field of health education which is becoming more and more important as we come to realize that some of our most serious problems of health and disease are linked with lifestyle and behaviour.[1]

Lifestyle and behaviour are influenced by many factors of which health education is only one. Education, however, is not only what we are formally taught in school, or what the state, health agencies, and health professionals try to teach us. From early childhood until old age we absorb from our environment messages related to health, some of them beneficial, others less so. This has been emphasized in regard to sex education in a recent book.[2]

When governments allow industry to pollute the environment, for example, the message is given that economic gain is more important than protection of health. When a person in a high government position—or an actor, or any other well-known personality—is depicted in photographs or on television holding or smoking a cigarette, the message given to the young is obvious. When an obese mother nibbles all the time at sweets and snacks, how can her children be expected to acquire a proper knowledge of oral hygiene or good dietary habits?

Are there any ethical issues in the attempts to educate and to learn as regards our health? Are we aware of the risks to our autonomy from the enormous power yielded by those controlling the mass communication media? Should we accept 'brain-washing' in this area? To what extent should we allow the state and other agencies to influence our life and behaviour? These and many other questions were discussed among a small group of scientists and we decided to seek contributions to answer them from representatives of many disciplines. The result was the present book.

The multidisciplinary composition of our team of authors is a guarantee of a representation of many points of view. There are many models or concepts of health and disease and therefore many models of health care which includes health education. It is obvious from the chapters of Section I of the book that we try to encompass many approaches. This section contains three chapters which examine the theoretical background of health education.

First, Downie examines some of the problems and assumptions common to any setting in which health education takes place. He discusses the nature of health itself and proceeds to make the important distinction between health promotion and health education. Campbell follows, discussing the difference between education and indoctrination. He accepts that persuasion is allowed, provided that the true picture of the various aspects of each topic is given. Gillon then examines health education within the framework of the four main moral principles of autonomy, beneficence, non-maleficence, and justice, and concludes that the same ethical dilemmas arise as in other aspects of medical care.

In Section II on Sociopolitical Issues, Gorovitz begins by discussing the impact of the increasing privatization of health care on the information given to the public. Experience in the United States shows the growing acceptability of medical advertising of both institutions and individuals. This should be a warning and a lesson for the European countries to keep health education as a non-commercial commitment.

Pattison and Player, with extensive experience in health education, examine its important sociopolitical implications. Using two case studies as examples, they identify the political pressures upon health education and conclude that state intervention should be accepted in spite of doubts as to its extent and emphasis.

Harlem then examines the role of organized medicine in health education. He describes the various Codes and Directives voted and propagated by the World Medical Association, and stresses the responsibility of both international and national medical associations in promoting scientifically based and socially acceptable messages of health education.

Flaysakier, with personal experience in medical journalism, suggests that lack of specialist knowledge of many of those involved in medical writing results in misinformation of the public and therefore in the breaking of ethical rules. He suggests that stricter ethical guidelines are necessary when health topics are described and projected in all types of communication media.

Section III is devoted to the issues related to the target groups of health education. The chapter by Garanis and myself examines the unconscious and hidden messages absorbed by very young children. These messages are contained not only in our conscious attempts to educate but also in all our acts and in our behaviour. All those in the environment of young children should, therefore, be aware that everything they do or say constitutes a hidden curriculum.

Downie and Fyfe describe the necessary criteria for inclusion of health education in a school curriculum in order to avoid ethical pitfalls. They suggest that the important criteria are the knowledge base, methods which respect the person, and the likely reasons for health education.

The next chapter concerns more specific issues of the ethics of health education, with Tountas writing on the relationship between health education and self-care or self-help. Is there any justification for support of self-care and if so what are the dilemmas in deciding between supporting autonomy, which is related to self-care, and allocation of resources which is inevitably a function of the state.

A book on the Ethics of Health Education could not be complete without a chapter on the problems which have recently emerged from the spread of AIDS with all the attendant psychological, social, and legal problems. This multitude of questions and dilemmas is described and discussed by Eisenberg.

Nutrition, including drinking habits, is another important aspect of lifestyle and behaviour. Health education related to these two important aspects creates ethical dilemmas which are explored by Riis.

The meaning of positive and negative mental health is discussed by Atkinson. She points out the important differences between physical and mental as well as social health in the field of health education, emphasizing the great ethical dilemmas arising when any 'health educator' attempts to engage in activities in this area.

This book is addressed to—and we hope will be read and found useful by—many persons belonging not only to the health sciences and professions but also to others such as lawyers, philosophers, sociologists, and political decision-makers. The importance of sensitizing and involving this last group in health education in its widest sense has been stressed recently.[3,4]

It was necessary, therefore, to include chapters and information which to many experts will appear elementary. My experience in the field of medical ethics, particularly in Europe, however, is that, with the exception of some of the advanced countries (in the west and the north of Europe), there is still a disturbing lack of interest and sensitivity for this field. A recent example is that, at a meeting organized by the European Office of the World Health Organization on The Ethics of Clinical Research, there were only two representatives from Eastern European countries and only one from the southern countries.

This volume on ethical issues in health education is an attempt to stimulate discussion of a part of medical ethics which so far has been very little explored, although it is becoming increasingly important. The book is based on experience in developed countries, but clearly many of the problems raised are shared, and will increasingly be faced, by those in the developing world as well. It is a vast subject and to cover all aspects in one book would be an impossible task. We have tried, therefore, simply to suggest areas of interest and concern that deserve to be more fully and thoughtfully studied and discussed.

REFERENCES

1. World Health Organization. *Education for Health: A Manual on Health Education in Primary Health Care*. Geneva: WHO, 1988.
2. Massey, D.E. *School Sex Education—Why, What and How?* London: Family Planning Association, 1988.

3. Rodmell, S. and Watt, Alison (eds.). *Politics of Health Education*. London: Routledge and Kegan Paul, 1986.
4. Research Unit in Health and Behavioural Change. *Changing the Public Health*. Chichester: Wiley, 1989.

SECTION I

THEORETICAL BACKGROUND

CHAPTER 1

Ethics in Health Education: An Introduction

R. S. DOWNIE

SUMMARY

In this short introductory chapter I examine some of the problems and assumptions which are common to any setting in which health education takes place. I will begin by discussing the nature of health itself. I will then look at the relationships between health education and medical practice and between health education and health promotion. Finally, I will consider briefly who are the health educators.

INTRODUCTION

In this book health education will be discussed from different points of view and the ethical problems it raises will be examined in various settings. In this brief introductory chapter I shall look at some of the problems and assumptions which are common to any setting in which health education takes place, beginning with the nature of health itself.

WHAT IS HEALTH?

The literature of health education tends nowadays to have a complex view of the concept of health and to distinguish various elements within it.

The first of those is often called 'negative health', or the absence of ill-health. 'Ill-health' itself is a complex notion comprising disease, illness, handicap, injury, and other related ideas. These overlapping concepts can be linked if they are seen on the model of abnormal, unwanted or incapacitating states of a biological system.[1,2]

Secondly, the idea of 'positive health' has more recently appeared in published reports. The origins of this idea are in the definition of health to be found in the preamble to the Constitution of the World Health Organization (WHO).

Ethics in Health Education
Edited by S. Doxiadis. ©1990 John Wiley & Sons Ltd

'Health is a state of complete physical, mental and social well-being, and not merely the absence of disease or infirmity.'[3]

It follows from this definition that 'well-being' is an important ingredient in positive health.

A third idea in the concept of health is that of 'fitness'. Fitness in its most obvious sense refers to the state of someone's heart and lungs. To be fit in this sense is to have a place on a scale ranging from being able to climb stairs or run for a bus without getting out of breath to being able to run a marathon or climb Mount Everest. Fitness can also be used in a related but broader sense, which we might call the 'sociological' as opposed to the 'heart and lungs' sense. In the sociological sense of fitness a person is fit *for* some occupation or job. This means that people have the necessary health to enable them to perform the job or task adequately without, for example, too many days off work.

It is tempting to think of fitness as standing alongside well-being as a component in positive health. But this is a mistake; fitness can be seen as part of either the negative or the positive dimensions of health. One is healthy in the negative sense if one is not ill or diseased; analogously one can be fit in the negative sense if one can perform the tasks of daily life—stair-climbing, walking to and fro, luggage-lifting and so on—without undue physical stress. The analogue to positive well-being is the fitness which enables a person to swim, ride a bicycle, climb a hill and so on. Fitness, then, is best seen as a component of both negative and positive health rather than as a separate dimension to health.

The WHO definition refers to the 'mental and social' as well as to the physical. Nevertheless, the mental and social components of health are the poor relations of the health services and do not receive adequate attention in published reports or adequate funding from governments or research institutions. Moreover, to begin with mental health, it is certainly true that mental health is most often taken to be the absence of mental ill-health. In Chapter 13 Atkinson makes a case for the existence of a positive dimension to mental health. The danger of this is that it might encourage conformity or fitting in with prevailing social norms and attitudes, but she manages to suggest ways of looking at positive mental health which avoid this charge.

The idea of 'social well-being' is in fact just as obscure as that of mental well-being, although at first sight it does not seem to be a difficult notion. What does it mean? In one sense 'social well-being' refers to the skills and other abilities which enable us to form friendships and relate to other people in conversation and through the many different sorts of contacts which are part of ordinary social life. Sometimes these are called 'lifeskills', and the possession of them helps to create a sense of 'self-esteem' which is currently a fashionable concept in the literature of health education. Clearly, like fitness, social well-being in this sense can be graded on a scale from negative to positive. It is a property of individuals and refers to their ability to cope in a social context—hence 'social well-being' is an appropriate term.

But does it make sense to speak of 'social well-being' in a stricter sense—one which makes the well-being a characteristic of society itself, as distinct from the individuals who are in society? One way of making sense of this idea is to think of society not in terms of the individuals who make it up, but in terms of the institutions, practices, customs, political arrangements, social class relationships and so on, which give structure to the society. From this point of view people are related to each other by the structures of their society, and indeed part of their identity is created by these social structures. We could then evaluate a society in terms of the way in which its social structures tend to produce well-being in the people who belong to that society. Just as we sometimes praise the 'atmosphere' in a school or hospital as one of well-being, so the social structures of an entire society might be said to make for or detract from well-being.

Some theorists with firm attachments to empiricism might prefer to understand what I have said as referring to health determinants rather than health itself. For example, they might agree that a society with marked social class gradients and corresponding gradients in the distribution of ill-health is one with a tendency to create ill-health in individuals. Thus, in terms of this approach, if we speak of an 'unhealthy society' we are simply speaking metaphorically about the determinants, such as poor housing, diet and so on, that have helped to produce poor health states in individuals. Other thinkers might be prepared to extend language and to maintain that it is not a metaphor to characterize social relationships and structures as being themselves unhealthy. It is perhaps self-indulgent to pursue this theoretical question here.

It is not self-indulgent, however, to examine the relationship between health negatively and health positively conceived. Can we link the absence of ill-health and the presence of well-being in a single concept of health in the manner of the WHO definition? This is not a rarefied question because it affects the legitimate scope of health education. If well-being is a component in the concept of health then clearly health education has a much wider remit than it would otherwise have.

One important factor influencing this question is that ill-health and well-being cannot be related to each other as opposite poles on a linear scale. This approach has been tried by some theorists,[4] but it is not satisfactory, for it is logically possible (and not in fact uncommon) for someone to have poor physical health but a high state of well-being—as in the case of a terminal patient in a hospice who is supported by a caring staff and loving friends—or a good state of physical health but poor well-being—as in the case of someone who has no diseases or illnesses but lacks friends, a job, interests.

The fact that health (the absence of ill-health) and well-being cannot be related on a linear scale must raise the question of whether they are in fact two components of a single concept. It may be preferable and less confusing conceptually to think of them as two overlapping concepts rather than as a single concept with two dimensions. Thus the feeling of well-being that a person has after an invigorating swim can fairly be described as a 'glow of health', but the well-being or satisfaction that a person has after writing a chapter in a book, listening to a piece of music, or just playing an enjoyable game is less obviously related to the concept of health, and more obviously related to concepts such as 'enjoyment', 'happiness', etc. Again, the well-being that is created by moving someone to better housing is more obviously related to the concept of 'welfare' than to that of health. The conclusion is that while the concepts of health and well-being overlap they are distinct and cannot be combined into one concept.[1]

It does not of course follow from the fact that well-being is a different concept from health that health education has no bearing on it. To take analogous cases, a health educationist, indeed a doctor, might reasonably be concerned with the processes of aging, or with contraception. But neither getting older as such nor pregnancy constitutes ill-health. In other words, just as the legitimate activities of a doctor may be wider than coping with ill-health, so the legitimate activities of a health educationist may be wider than anything reasonably called 'health'. But what are the reasonable activities of health education?

HEALTH EDUCATION AND MEDICAL PRACTICE

At a very general level we can answer the question by a broad statement of aim:

> Health education is an activity aimed at restoring, maintaining, or enhancing the health of individuals and communities.

This definition is not adequate, however, for it provides at best a necessary and not a sufficient definition of health education. The definition as stated could apply to the work of the doctor. Doctors of course see themselves as health educators, but in their characteristic work they are concerned not with education but with treatment. How then can we distinguish the work of the health educator from that of the doctor?

There are various important differences in assumption and approach. To state these is not necessarily to state a preference for one or the other. The activities are complementary and overlap, and as has already been said, the doctor can at times act as a health educator. Nevertheless, there are differences. But before listing these we must first dispel one confusion.

It is sometimes suggested that medicine deals with scientific fact whereas health education deals with advice and exhortation: one deals with the 'is' and the other with the 'ought'. This is not true. Medicine is based on the sciences, but it also deals with advice and with prescriptions. Health education is likewise based on the biological and social sciences, but also advises and counsels. What then are the genuine differences?

First, medicine characteristically bypasses our rational minds and treats us as causal mechanisms. In other words, characteristic medical treatments are biochemical or surgical, whereas health education characteristically attempts to get us to understand our bodies and their environment. Secondly, medicine typically (but again by no means exclusively) stresses the curative or palliative, whereas health education stresses the preventive. Going along with the second distinction we might say, thirdly, that medicine stresses the doctor–patient or one-to-one relationship, whereas health education tends to have a broader societal perspective. Fourthly, and perhaps most fundamentally, medicine tends to be reductivist in its assumptions—this follows from the scientific study of disease processes on which it is based—whereas health education tends to be holistic in its assumptions.

Does it follow from these distinctions, if they contain at least some truth, that health education is in some way ethically superior to medicine? This by no means follows. If I break my leg I do not want advice and holistic treatment! In other words, there is a place for both approaches. What does follow is that health education gives rise to an acute set of ethical problems because it is interfering with lifestyle. It therefore requires considerable ethical justification. This point is stressed by Gillon in Chapter 3.

HEALTH EDUCATION AND HEALTH PROMOTION

The first attempt at a definition of health education which was offered at the beginning of the previous section did not succeed in distinguishing health education from medical practice. Neither did it distinguish health education from health promotion. Can the latter two be distinguished?[5]

This is not a question of finding some ingenious method of distinguishing two things that are essentially different (as one might attempt to devise a method to separate two chemical substances). It is a matter of reviewing the practices of health education and health promotion as described in the literature and *stipulating* a distinction which seems helpful.

Several possible ways of drawing the distinction are not satisfactory. It might be said that traditionally health education has been concerned with negative health, whereas health promotion is concerned with positive health. Now no doubt health education once had a mainly negative focus, but there is no reason why it should not be allowed to develop—it clearly has—and concern itself also with positive health. Indeed, more recent criticisms of health education are first that it does concern itself with positive health or well-being, and that this involves interference with people's lifestyles; and secondly that claims to have an expertise which entitles a health educationist to educate about well-being or happiness are bogus; there is no such expertise. These criticisms are discussed more fully by Downie and Fyfe in Chapter 9.

A second superficial contrast is to the effect that health education, like all true education, respects the autonomy of its recipients, whereas health promotion bypasses autonomy and sells health like a commodity. In this it might be said to resemble the advertisements for unhealthy products which it is opposing.[6] This point is discussed by Gorovitz in Chapter 4.

In reply to this argument we might question the premise that all true education respects autonomy. It might be maintained that autonomy is not something which everyone in fact possesses. People can be victims of all sorts of social processes and be lacking in power. It is quite unrealistic to regard all recipients of health education as autonomous. Education of any kind, whether concerned with health or not, must take into account the fact that people, young or old, must be 'empowered', and education is an important part of the process of empowerment. It must aim at creating or enhancing autonomy, but should not presuppose it. This issue is ethically important and must be examined in more detail. Is health education really 'education' or is it rather 'training', 'instruction', or even 'indoctrination'? Some of the issues here will be discussed in succeeding chapters, (notably by Campbell in Chapter 2), but it may be helpful to introduce them briefly here.

The criteria for calling an activity 'educational' have been worked out in much detail in the many writings of R. S. Peters,[7,8] and it is illuminating to look at health education in the light of the distinctions he drew between 'training' or 'instruction' on the one hand and 'education' on the other.[9] It should be said that Peters developed the distinctions in slightly different ways in different works and what is offered here is, therefore, more of a paraphrase of his distinctions than an expression of any one way in which he drew them.

The first and most important criterion is that something worthwhile or valuable for its own sake must be passed on in any activity which is properly to be called education. It is obvious that Fagan's class in picking pockets in Dicken's *Oliver Twist*, while it may have been training, could not be regarded as education, because it was actually harmful to others. There are also neutral activities which may count as 'training' but are not 'education' in terms of Peters' distinction. A student, for example, can be trained to give an intravenous injection, but this is not education although the technique when learned can be used to help a patient. In terms of this distinction teaching on health may or may not count as 'education'. To the extent that we concentrate on the practical uses of health education we are thinking of it as training for a further end—such as cutting down expenditure on health care, improving the efficiency of industry, reducing the number of days off work, and so on. But to the extent that we stress the intrinsic value of the human biology and behavioural sciences involved in health education, and the intrinsic value of health itself as a component in a good or flourishing human life, we are seeing it as a part of education.

The second criterion which any activity must satisfy if it is to be educational is that it must have wide cognitive perspectives. Thus, activities such as science, history, literature, and so on are central to education, not only because they are valuable in themselves but also because they may deepen and widen one's understanding of other matters. Imagine, for example, a historian of the French

Revolution who was surprised when he was told that a study of this period led people to think of such matters as social justice, and said that he was just interested in 'the facts'. It might be more appropriate to say of such a person that he had been 'trained' as a historian than that he had been educated as one. In terms of this criterion we can again look at health education in different ways, depending on how it is taught and at what level. If it is taught as a set of 'tips' for healthy living then it is instruction or training, but it can be taught at a higher level with wide cognitive perspectives. Several chapters in this book illustrate some of the wide cognitive perspectives of health education. In Chapter 11, for example, Eisenberg places the problem of AIDS in wide biological and cultural perspectives; Pattison and Player in Chapter 5 are concerned with social and political perspectives; and Doxiadis and Garanis in Chapter 8 give us insights into the development of the young child. Indeed, the book as a whole is intended to locate health education in the broad context of ethical thinking.

The third criterion which any educational activity must satisfy, besides being valuable in itself and related to other activities thought valuable, is that those engaged in it must come to care about what they are doing. Suppose that students have completed courses in biology or literature (activities which are valuable in themselves and have wide cognitive perspectives) but thereafter show no interest in these subjects. We might say that they have been highly trained or instructed but, if they do not care about what they have studied, they are not educated. In terms of this criterion health education can count as part of education. Indeed, one of the main points of health education is to encourage people to care about their health, to view health as a value in its own right regardless of its usefulness.

Fourthly, education implies that a person's whole outlook has been transformed—it involves 'wholeness'—whereas training suggests a competence of more limited scope. In terms of this criterion health education can count as education. Indeed, in terms of this criterion it does better than many subjects traditionally regarded as part of education. Health is such a central aspect of human existence that if someone can be brought to value his own health and that of his community in the context of the commercial and environmental threats to it, his outlook will really have been transformed. Education, as distinct from training, has to do with opening out, with 'educing', with releasing and liberating (as Rita found in the film and play *Educating Rita*). This is one realistic possibility for health education, and one which makes it ethically worthwhile.

Fifthly, it follows from the previous point that the educator must employ different methods from the trainer or instructor. It is consistent with training or instruction, for example, to use methods based on fear, threats, indoctrination, or hidden persuasion. By contrast, the educator must always use person-respecting methods. As Campbell stresses in Chapter 2, education must encourage critical thought and must be a two-way process.

But, as I have already stressed, we must not exaggerate the extent to which human being are autonomous, rational, and critical thinkers. In view of the political and commercial power of the anti-health forces in society exposed by Pattison and Player (Chapter 5), health must be presented in as attractive a way as possible or health education will fail totally. If health educators insist on confining themselves strictly to the rational, critical approach to education, then it is preferable to depict health education as an element within a larger health promotion movement concerned with legislative change, fiscal reform, and the mobilization of community interests as well as education narrowly conceived.

The tension between the ethical requirement to be person-respecting in methods and the practical necessity to be effective is addressed from an interesting point of view in Chapter 10 by Tountas. The growth of self-care groups concerned with every conceivable malady and involving both the sufferers and their relatives has been a notable development during the last decade. These movements avoid the charge of paternalism commonly still made against every branch of health care, including health education. Apart from ethical considerations, self-care movements seem to be effective within their limits, although they may benefit from a professional health educator to advise and facilitate. Advising and facilitating is indeed an important role for health education.

Let me now sum up this discussion as to whether health education is really 'education'. The argument has been that health education can be genuinely educative. In terms of its content and its method it can pass on something worthwhile or valuable for its own sake, it can have a wide cognitive perspective, it can encourage its students to care about health and so transform their outlook, it can use person-respecting methods, although it is important that these methods should be appropriate for young children as stressed in Chapters 8 and 9, or for those at risk from anti-health movements.

I now return to the question of the definition of health education and its relationship to health promotion from which I began this section. What has emerged is that while it is not difficult to distinguish health education from the practice of medicine in terms of aim and method, it is much less easy to draw distinctions between health education and health promotion. If we think of health promotion as comprising all those activities which are aimed at preventing ill-health and furthering positive health then we can think of health education as an important sub-set of this. A positive definition of health education can now be suggested.[1]

> Health education is an activity aimed at preventing ill-health and furthering positive health through creating an understanding of the human body and its workings, through the provision of information about health service and access to them, and through creating understanding of national or local policies and environmental processes which may be detrimental to health.

It follows from this definition that health education is indeed education in the fullest sense. But it also follows that health education cannot be widely effective on its own but needs to be supplemented by and seen in the wider perspective of health promotion if it is to be effective. This approach to health education and health promotion is in accord with the WHO account (1984).[10]

The relationship between health education, health promotion, and prevention which is here proposed can be represented as shown in Figure 1.

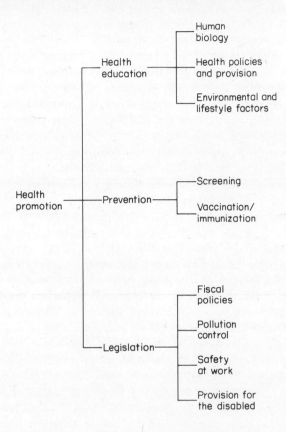

Figure 1   Relationship between health education, health promotion, and prevention.

WHO ARE THE HEALTH EDUCATORS?

It will be clear from the definition of health education proposed, as well as from the varied backgrounds and professional interests of the authors of the chapters which follow, that a large number of different professions are involved in health education. It is therefore easy to forget that health education is itself a profession and that there are national health education bodies. In the United Kingdom these were established after the Cohen Report.[11] Recently in the United Kingdom there has been an increased political interest in health education and promotion (the two are not clearly distinguished in the official mind) and now most health authorities employ health education or promotion officers. From a national point of view, in the United Kingdom responsibility for health education is vested in the Health Education Authority (England), the Scottish Health Education Group, the Welsh Health Promotion Authority, and the Northern Ireland Health Promotion Unit.

The role of health education officers differs from that of school teachers. In other words, health education officers are less concerned with health education directly than with enabling other professionals to fulfil their possibilities as health educators. They operate at a second-order level to assist a host of other professionals in varied spheres to acquire the skills and knowledge involved in health education. Likewise, the national bodies, while they may at times be involved in national campaigns to promote health, see their major role as being that of facilitating campaigns at a grass-roots level. This may be the most effective use of their resources, [12,13] but it is also ethically the best approach, for it involves local people in local problems and is therefore a 'bottom up' rather than a 'top down' approach. This is an approach which is consistent with the principle of respect for autonomy.

Thus most health education is carried out, not by professional health education officers, but by other health and education professionals. This has drawbacks, both practically and ethically. It is all too easy for health professionals, especially those like doctors who are in positions of high status and power in the community, to think of education as something which it is easy to carry out—all that is necessary is to tell patients what they need to do to maintain their health. It is easy to underestimate the problems faced by the powerless in society in rejecting anti-health forces. The result of insensitive or ill-informed attempts at health education can be distressing to the victims of anti-health forces and can create attitudes hostile to healthy lifestyles. Moralizing is not educating.

The chapters in this book are not uncritical of health education and certainly show an awareness of the ethical problems in its many domains. Nevertheless, we hope that our wide-ranging and open-ended discussions will encourage international cooperation in ethically principled health education.

REFERENCES

1. Downie, R.S., Fyfe, C. and Tannahill, A. *Health Promotion: Models and Values*. Oxford: Oxford University Press, 1990.
2. Seedhouse, D. *Health: The Foundations of Achievement*. Chichester: John Wiley, 1986.
3. World Health Organization. Constitution. New York, 1946.
4. Catford, J.C. Positive health indicators towards a new information base for health promotion. *Comm Med* 1983; **5**: 125-132.
5. Doxiadis, S. (ed.) *Ethical Dilemmas in Health Promotion*. Chichester: John Wiley & Sons, 1987.
6. Williams, G. Health promotion—caring concern or slick salesmanship? *J Med Ethics* 1984; **10**: 191–195.
7. Peters, R.S. (ed.) *The Philosophy of Education*. Oxford: Oxford University Press, 1973.
8. Peters, R.S. *Ethics and Education*. London: Allen and Unwin, 1966.

9. Calman, K.C. and Downie, R.S. Education and training in medicine. *Med Ed* 1988; **22**: 488–491.
10. WHO Health Promotion: A discussion document on the concept and principles. Copenhagen: World Health Organization, 1984.
11. Ministry of Health. Health Education. Report of the Joint Committee of the Central and Scottish Health Services Councils. Chairman, Lord Cohen of Birkenhead. London: Her Majesty's Stationery Office, 1964.
12. Tones, B.K. Training needs for health education. *J Inst Hlth Ed* 1977; **15(1)**: 22–29.
13. Tones, B.K. Effective education and health. In *Health Education in Schools*. Cawley, J., David, K., and Williams, T. (eds.). London: Harper and Row, 1981.

CHAPTER 2

Education or Indoctrination? The Issue of Autonomy in Health Education

ALASTAIR V. CAMPBELL

SUMMARY

How is a distinction to be drawn between education and indoctrination in health education? This issue is explored by clarifying the meaning of the terms 'education', 'health', and 'indoctrination', and by relating this discussion to the moral principle of safeguarding the autonomy of the individual in health care. It is concluded that powerfully persuasive methods may be used, including those which can bring about political change, provided there is no concealment or distortion of the relevant facts. A recent controversy in the United Kingdom concerning the safety of eggs and soft cheese provides an illustrative epilogue to the general issues raised.

INTRODUCTION

Is health education morally justifiable? This may seem at first sight such a ridiculous question that only a philosopher would think of asking it. Surely anything which can encourage people to have a greater concern for their own health and to avoid health-destructive behaviour must be morally praiseworthy! Yet, in reality the issue is not so clear-cut. In the first place, there are a number of different reasons for the current enthusiasm (not always matched by funding) for government sponsored health education. For some politicians and health administrators it seems to promise economies in the health budget by reducing, even if only marginally, the burden of ill-health created by smoking, alcohol abuse, and so on. Others see it as a means of protecting the community from harm—for example, by reducing the number of drunken drivers or by controlling the spread of AIDS. Others again see it solely in terms of the gains to the individuals or groups receiving the education, arguing that any gain in self-determination is itself a gain in health, since health is autonomy.[1] These reasons are not of course mutually exclusive, but the approach to health

Ethics in Health Education
Edited by S. Doxiadis. ©1990 John Wiley & Sons Ltd

education will be markedly different depending on the goal sought and it is only in the last approach that the protection of autonomy of the individual is regarded as paramount.

A second problem is that the very term 'health education' lacks clarity of definition. Does it encompass the whole range of activities sometimes described as 'health promotion', in which the techniques of persuasion developed in mass advertising are fully used? Or should it be restricted to the kind of introduction to facts and theories normally associated with education in school or university? If the latter, more purist, approach proves ineffective in altering attitudes and behaviour, is there a moral imperative to use more persuasive techniques or are we thereby abandoning education for indoctrination?

Thirdly, who is to determine priorities in this field, and what is the nature of the 'health' which is sought as an outcome? Is it enough that the incidence of avoidable illness and accidents be reduced, or should more idealistic goals like the World Health Organization's 'complete physical, mental and social well-being' be sought through educational means? Should health education do more than change the attitudes and behaviour of individuals? Should it seek to re-educate or reform whole societies?

This morass of unanswered questions makes a simple assessment of the value of health education impossible. I shall not, therefore, attempt such a task in this chapter, but will restrict the discussion to one (arguably central) issue: the relationship between health education and the moral value of respecting the autonomy of the individual. After looking more closely at the nature of this value, I shall conclude that to safeguard autonomy we are entitled to employ powerfully persuasive methods of influencing both individual attitudes and political policies in health care. Nevertheless, the need to make health education effective does not justify the abandoning of education for indoctrination. My discussion will fall into two parts. In the first I shall discuss how education in general relates to the value of autonomy; in the second I shall explore approaches to health education which are effective but not merely manipulative and paternalistic.

AUTONOMY AND EDUCATION

It is to the philosopher Immanuel Kant that we owe the first major formulation of the moral value of the autonomy of the individual. Kant argued that 'freedom of the will' was the supreme principle of moral action. Actions did not gain their moral worth from consequences alone, but from the fact that they were freely chosen by moral agents acting out of respect for the moral law. Such moral agents (or 'rational beings' as Kant called them) should never be treated as mere means to some end, however worthy. They themselves must be given the opportunity to participate in such decisions, to become 'self-legislating members of a rational kingdom of ends.[2] It should be noted that Kant was not advocating 'individual freedom' in any simple sense—he was no mere laissez-faire libertarian. On the contrary, for him the rationality of the agent's choices was paramount, and if one failed to act on the basis of some rational principle, then the action was in effect not free at all, but simply the outcome of irrational forces. The moral—or immoral—action stemmed from a choice to follow—or fail to follow—the rational principles which formed the basis of all moral action. Thus *autonomy* in Kant's theory consisted in willed obedience to the moral law: *heteronomy* consisted in following preferences or prudential considerations. The autonomous moral agent would obey the 'categorical imperatives' of genuine moral action: the heteronomous moral agent would be swayed by inclination and preference, following the 'hypothetical imperatives' (*if* you want x, then *do* y) which would ensure their satisfaction. In Kantian ethics, pure duty must always prevail over the pursuit of pleasure or of personal gratification.

In more modern discussions of moral autonomy there has been a tendency to move away from Kant's heavy stress on rationality and on duty, and to emphasize instead the integrative aspects of personal identity, whereby the maturing individual forms a coherent set of goals or values which shape both the emotional and the rational aspects of decision-making. In such formulations 'respect for persons' becomes the shorthand formula for what was described in Kantian terms as 'treating all rational beings as ends in themselves', but preferences and desires are also allowed for in this respect for other persons. We give to others the freedom to shape their personal lives according to their own goals and we expect the same respect for ourselves.[3] But even in this looser modern formulation there remains the concern that autonomy is under hazard from both internal and external sources. For Kant, 'bondage of the will' consisted in allowing the emotions to hold sway over the clear dictates of duty coming from the reason alone. A less rationalist, more personalist approach would be more concerned with the detrimental affect on decision-making of emotional bias, inadequate information, and false beliefs. Thus, in *The Value of Life* John Harris describes autonomy as:

> ... 'critical self-determination in which the agent strives to make decisions which are as little marred by defects in reason, information or control as she can make them...'[4]

We note in this description the key terms 'critical' and 'control'. These both imply a measure of self-scrutiny and emotional integration which does not come naturally to us but is the product of both emotional and intellectual maturation. Similarly, Richard Lindley, in his book discussing both personal and political autonomy,[5] identifies both a *cognitive* and *conative* hazard to autonomy. The former stems from the failure to use one's reason actively to establish the reliability of the beliefs upon which decisions are made, while the latter stems from an irrational tendency to act inconsistently with one's expressed preferences in life. Thus we can perceive the nature of autonomy more clearly by noting its absence in such poorly controlled actions. Autonomy is possible only when we are able to act consistently and in a reasonably well-informed manner.

We are now in a position to relate the nature of education in general to the fostering of moral autonomy. The relationship is clearly a very close one. According to R.S. Peters, education is 'initiation into what is worthwhile with the provision that what has been transmitted has been taught in a morally unobjectionable way.'[6] In a later essay,[7] Peters elaborates this definition by stressing that the aims of education and the procedures of education cannot really be separated. If the principal aim of education is to produce the 'educated man', then the process of education must be one which depends upon the fostering of autonomy, self-origination, individual choice, and individual difference. Whatever content is included in the activity of education, it is the method by which the content is communicated that determines the successful outcome.

The connection between education and individual autonomy comes out even more strongly in Glenn Langford's assertion that 'to become educated is to learn to be a person.'[8] Langford expounds the concept of 'person' in terms of the nature of human consciousness. Persons, he claims, have a developed capacity to structure the world by means of concepts and thereby to pursue plans based on chosen ends. It is this capacity which education seeks to develop fully, by enhancing the individual's ability to assess evidence, test the truth of beliefs, and refine both intellectual and non-intellectual skills relevant to appropriate goal-directed actions.

In light of these philosophical accounts of the nature of education, it hardly needs stating that methods which attempt to impose fixed attitudes and beliefs upon individuals and which fail to promote their capacities for independent judgment and choice are profoundly anti-educational. It is the encouragement of independent thought which sets education apart from training, social conditioning and, above all, indoctrination. As R.M. Hare puts it:

> 'The educator is waiting and hoping all the time for those whom he is educating to start *thinking*... The indoctrinator, on the other hand, is watching for signs of trouble, and ready to intervene to suppress it when it appears...'[9]

Then how are we to understand 'health education'—as genuine education or as indoctrination, as an enhancement of autonomy or as merely the substitution of one heteronomy for another, the paternalistic beneficence of the 'health expert'?

INDOCTRINATION, PERSUASION, AND HEALTH EDUCATION

What is Health Education?

In considering this question we are faced at once by the complexity of the definitions which are offered by those advocating health education. Thompson begins with what may seem a relatively simple definition:

'A range of educational activities, whether directed at individuals or communities, which are concerned with the prevention of disease or injury, as well as the promotion of positive health.'[10]

But as he elaborates his definition, in terms of four models—medical, educational, community development, and sociopolitical—it becomes clear that a very wide sweep of activities has been included, ranging from the simple communication of medical facts through a *formative (not merely informative)* educational approach to the transformation of society and the control of vested interests. In similar fashion, Draper and colleages [11] delineate three types of health education. The first two are concerned with education about human health and about available resources for health care, but the third deals with the whole environment within which health choices are made and with the national policies which influence that environment. An illustrative example may be taken from cigarette smoking. Type 1 education would warn individuals of the health hazards of smoking and seek to change their habits; type 2 would inform people of resources available for the early detection and therapy of smoking-related diseases; but type 3 health education would raise much wider issues arising from the 'tobacco smoking environment', such as the stress which leads to the need for tranquillization by tobacco, the role of multinational companies in advertising and exerting political pressure, and the revenue aspects both for governments and for the media advertising the product. In light of these wider sociopolitical issues the authors argue that health education must be much more than simply telling people to 'adopt healthy lifestyles' or 'be responsible'. Rather, it must confront the 'religion' of modern society, 'our preoccupation with economic growth':

'... health education should, in the last analysis, contribute to developing a society based on an economy that promotes health and wellbeing rather than one that too often pursues "wealth" at the expense of health.'[11]

It is evident that the more we consider the nature of health education, the more we must consider the complex question of the nature of health itself. As Coutts and Hardy have pointed out,[12] traditional approaches to health education depended on the idea that medical science could be used to ensure *prevention* of disease. On the basis of this 'medical model' a stress is laid on the communication of information by medical experts about health hazards, improvements in diet and hygiene, and protection against communicable diseases. This traditional model is certainly not obsolete, as the problem of the prevention of the spread of AIDs—discussed by Eisenberg in Chapter 11—graphically illustrates, but it is clearly inadequate. An individual's health is not ensured merely by the avoidance of disease, but also depends crucially upon his or her own attitudes to life and on the extent to which society promotes or inhibits individual well-being and the ability for full self-development. Thus Seedhouse[13] aptly describes health as 'the foundations for achievement' and he stresses that such achievement is as much mental as physical:

> 'Education for health is work for wholeness. It is not just to do with physical functioning, it is at least equally to do with the mental life of the person ... work for health in its full and proper sense is work toward laying the foundations for full human flourishing.'

In an approach like that of Seedhouse, education for health entails a full respect for the autonomy of individuals. Indeed Seedhouse sees as an inevitable concomitant of effective health education the removal of health policy from the domain of medical science and the fostering of an informed and articulate public, which will seek political change to ensure a healthier and more humane society. Tones (who supports similar ideals) provides us with an example of the antithesis of this approach in the following definition by Baric:

> 'In societal terms health is defined as a state of optimum capacity of an individual for the effective performance of the roles and tasks for which he has been socialised.'[14]

Undoubtedly a concern for individual autonomy commits us to a more revolutionary view of health education than that espoused by Baric. Adaptation to a social role could mean for the individual a serious restriction of potential and a loss of any sense of personal identity and worth, outcomes which would be seen (by most philosophers at least) as health-destructive. On the other hand, too much stress on individual development could also result in the loss of another component of human well-being—a sense of commitment to the human community as a whole. This aspect is described, in rather high-flown language, by the moral theologian, Peter Baelz, as follows:

> 'Health care is an aspect of human caring, caring for oneself as a human being with a personal identity to discover and develop, caring for one another within a community of responsible and responsive fellow beings.'[15]

If we espouse such a complex concept of health, one which encompasses both avoidance of disease and development of positive health and which stresses a communal as well as a personal dimension, then there clearly can be no single model for health education. It must embrace a wide variety of strategies for change of the kind summarized by Thompson[10] and by Draper and colleagues[11], crossing the boundaries between education of the individual, development of community awareness, and facilitation of political change. But what then are the methods which are ethically acceptable in such a broad approach to health education? It is clear that emotional and attitudinal change is aimed for, and not simply the provision of relevant information. Is such an approach different in kind from the persuasive techniques used in advertising or in political propaganda? Is propaganda *for* health any less objectionable than propaganda in general? And how do we distinguish health education from health indoctrination?

The Nature of Indoctrination

Like education, indoctrination seeks to induce change in the individual. Then how are they to be distinguished from one another? Classically, indoctrination has been understood as a way of inculcating unquestioning adherence to religious beliefs, particularly by influencing children (Jesuistical style) from an impressionable age. In the words of John Dryden:

'By education most have been mis-led;
So they believe because they were so bred.
The priest confirms what nursery began,
And thus the child imposes on the man.'

But indoctrination is now understood neither to be an inevitable concomitant of religious education nor to be confined to it. According to Snook,[16] the content of what is communicated is not the critical factor, nor even is the method as such—for a skilled indoctrinator could put on a convincing appearance of impeccable educational method as, for example, with some of the promotional material produced by some drug companies. The critical discriminator, in Snook's view, is the *intention* of the indoctrinator. Only if there is the *intention to impart beliefs regardless of the evidence* can we be sure that the activity is indoctrination and not education.

Thus the essence of indoctrination is that it deliberately ignores an individual's ability to reason in its commitment to the spreading of 'irrefutable' beliefs as widely as possible. As Smart points out,[17] the indoctrinator regards his subjects as mere means, not as ends in themselves. They are to be the passive recipients of a fixed set of ideas. This point is made still more powerfully by John Wilson, who locates the moral unacceptability of indoctrination in its tendency to diminish rationality:

'To put it dramatically: there is always hope so long as the mind remains free, however much our behaviour may be forced or our feelings conditioned. But if we occupy the inner citadel of thought and language, then it is difficult to see how a person can develop or regain rationality except by a long and arduous course of treatment.'[18]

Then what do we say of approaches to health education which go far beyond the simple inculcation of facts to the formation of attitudes and the challenging of the 'religion' of materialism? In a hard-hitting article,[19] Williams has claimed that broad definitions of health education are at best so bland and vague as to be meaningless, and at worst justifications of parternalistic interventions in the lives of others on the grounds that thereby 'better health' will be achieved. Noting a move towards a 'hard sell' approach to health promotion, Williams suggests that it is time that we asked the same questions of the 'slick salesman of health' that we would ask any salesman: what's in it for the salesman? What is he actually offering for sale and do we really need it? Does it do what it is claimed to do and could it do us more harm than good? Thus Williams wants the principle of *caveat emptor* introduced to health promotional activities—and she believes that the buyer has much to beware of, especially when there is pressure on health professionals from governments to 'get results'. In such an atmosphere, avers Williams, it is inevitable that the subtleties of individual choice are ignored in favour of some measurable behavioural changes in large groups.

The conclusion which Williams reaches on the basis of this radical critique of health promotion may be quoted in full, since it represents one possible conclusion of this chapter. In her view, the truly committed health educator should have no truck with health promotional methods:

'Health promotion, like advertising campaigns, cannot hope to do more than induce superficial change, which is susceptible to the next round of gimmicks or hard sell. Long-term commitment to sensible health behaviour . . . is needed if we are to improve health, and this is a function of education not promotion. Indeed, the very activity of hard-sell promotion is in direct conflict with the rational decision-making and personal autonomy which are central to educational, long-term goals, and the two cannot co-exist.'[19]

On Being or Not Being Persuaded

Williams' purist solution to the problem of this chapter is attractive in its simplicity, and much of her criticism of current promotional activities cannot be easily refuted. However, the contrast she draws between health education and health promotion is not really as absolute as she claims. All education contains *some* element of persuasion, even if it is no more than that of persuading people to pay attention to the issues being discussed. The fact that education is wholly committed to the fostering of autonomy and rationality does not in itself rule out the use of methods which go beyond a simple rational appeal. But one can agree with Williams that the enhancement of individual autonomy must always be the ultimate goal. (We are here close to the famous principle enunciated by the Reverend Rowland Hill that he did not see why the devil should not have all the good tunes.) It is also unfortunate that Williams seems to overlook the concern expressed in type 3 health education regarding the climate of expectations and the political structures within which people decide about their lifestyles. There is thus a dangerous naiveté in her faith in purely rationalistic and individualist methods of health education.

How then is health education to be an effective antidote to the hidden persuaders and an effective counterforce to commercial and political health-destructive forces, without itself being corrupted by the methods it employs? I must first stress that I raise this question in the context only of adult education—Doxiadis and Garanis (Chapter 8) and Downie and Fyfe (Chapter 9) will later in this volume discuss health education directed toward children and young people. In dealing with adults who are themselves the recipients of a bombardment of advertising for the 'good life' of material possessions, there can be no excuse for poorly produced and unsophisticated education programmes. It must, of course, be accepted that the battle for people's attention will always be an unequal one. No government or voluntary organization can possibly match the revenue spent by commercial interests in marketing their products. However, scruples against attempts to match their style of promotion reveal a confusion in thinking. Persuasive techniques which present facts about health hazards or health opportunities in a truthful and balanced way can enhance rather than diminish autonomy, since they draw attention to a range of choices of which the individual may not have been aware. For example, an attractively presented programme about food, nutrition, and the relationship between diet and health, may well alter people's purchasing habits and create a whole new demand for products not previously available from the mass producers of foodstuffs. The purchasers in this situation have had their autonomy increased by methods which altered their awareness of the choices open to them.

Such an approach to health education becomes indoctrination *only* if the presenters of a health issue deliberately distort the available facts or conceal ambiguities in the evidence in order to persuade the audience to accept their conclusions without question. Even then, however, most adults can readily tell when they are being energetically persuaded to adopt certain lifestyles or change certain behaviours, and because they are aware of it, they are thereby able to decide for themselves whether the persuader is to be believed. What is much harder to spot and to protect oneself against are manipulative measures of persuasion which bring about a change of attitude without the subject being fully aware of what is happening. Subliminal projection of messages during a programme ostensibly about something else is an extreme example of this, but there also exists a grey area in which the message is covert or partly explicit, but then given powerful reinforcement by symbols of safety, power, or success. It is at this point that an argument for 'effectiveness' in health education must be subjected to Williams' critical questioning. If autonomy is the paramount value in health education, then it must totally eschew any method which hides the intention of the educator, distorts the evidence in order to persuade, or uses any other wholly manipulative methods.

Finally, if health education is to enhance autonomy in the health sphere on any large scale, then it itself must be totally free from the control of special interest groups, both commercial and party political. There exists already within the health services a concept of professional autonomy, which (when effective and not merely self-serving) sets the patient's well-being and freedom of choice at the centre of the stage and resists all pressure to conform to commercial or political expediency. Whether such professional autonomy can continue to coexist with the new pressures to effectiveness in preventive medicine is the subject of the next chapter in this book. From the point of view of this more general discussion, however, the issue is relevant to all those responsible for funding, planning, and delivering health educational programmes. There will be no effective health education of the kind which empowers people to seek a more health-enhancing society, if politically inexpedient or commercially embarrassing facts about current destructive trends cannot be freely discussed. If, for example, there are still aspects of the marketing of food products which encourage health hazardous diets, then it is the function of the health educationist to make these as widely known as possible. Similarly, if economic policies creating high levels of unemployment are significantly related to the ill-health of sections of the population, then it should not be regarded as party political to inform the public of this correlation. For health education to be genuinely educational its independence and total commitment to factual accuracy must be beyond question.

This is perhaps a rather naive hope for health education, as naive as that expressed by Williams in her plea for purity of educational method. Yet Wilson was surely right in his insistence on the defence of the 'inner citadel of thought and language' against all false educators. Should it be the case that health education is in danger of becoming the Newspeak of commercial and political powers, then 1984, though chronologically past, still lies threateningly before us, and, in the pressure to serve the supposed 'common good', individual autonomy will be irretrievably lost.

EPILOGUE: EGGS AND SOFT CHEESE—A CAUTIONARY TALE

The issues explored in this chapter may be aptly illustrated by a controversy sparked off in the United Kingdom by some remarks by a junior health minister, Mrs Edwina Currie, which subsequently cost her her job. On 3 December 1988 Mrs Currie stated that 'most egg production in this country [the UK] is sadly infected by salmonella.' Her remarks were founded on good scientific evidence, but, as a House of Commons Select Committee has reported,[20] they were an exaggeration of the facts available to the Ministry at the time and caused unnecessary alarm. In September 1988 the Government's chief medical officer had issued a warning to food processors about salmonella in eggs[21] and there had since been ample documentation in the medical press of an increase of epidemic proportions of *Salmonella enteritidis* PT4 found in chicken carcasses and eggs.[22-24] In the period from 1981 to 1988 notified cases in England and Wales increased from 392 to 10 554 and there was a similar increase in Scotland.[25] The public reaction to Mrs Currie's statement was one of alarm and confusion, and there was a slump in the market for eggs and poultry. This in turn enraged the producers and, with the National Farmers' Union threatening civil action to recover their members' financial losses and a general air of confusion emanating from both the Ministry of Health and the Ministry of Agriculture, Fisheries and Food, Mrs Currie was persuaded to resign. In the rising tide of public disquiet about food safety, the British Government took a series of steps designed to reassure the public of their concern for their health. A House of

Commons Select Committee investigated the whole affair, tougher legislation was introduced to control the production of both eggs and poultry,[26] a new committee on Microbiological Food Safety was established,[25] and a pamphlet advising the public on safe food handling and cooking procedures was promised.

But, scarcely was the dust settling on the 'curried eggs' controversy, when a fresh announcement by the Department of Health (10 February 1989) warned the public of the dangers of listeria contamination of soft cheeses. This caused consternation in Britain's Common Market partners who produce such cheeses— the French press reminded its readers of the perfidy of the English at Agincourt! The cheese producers accused the United Kingdom Government of smokescreen tactics designed to divert attention from the controversy over eggs and the major retail chains expressed anger at such scaremongering. The British public was left, as a *Lancet* editorial pointed out,[25] with the uneasy impression that there was nothing left to eat that might not carry undeclared risks of infection!

The most salutary lesson to be learned from both of these controversies is that commercial and political pressures will inevitably have a detrimental effect on the major aim of health education—that of enabling all members of society to make responsible choices about their own health. It has now been revealed that as early as 1987 the Ministry of Health was aware that 60% of raw chickens from retail outlets were contaminated, mostly with salmonella,[26] but even when the Chief Medical Officer issued his warning in September 1988, it was not effective in informing the *consumers* of infected poultry products. That outcome awaited Mrs Currie's politically injudicious and exaggerated statement. A similar situation existed with knowledge of listeria contamination: a year before the public announcement, the Department of Health knew that 10% of soft cheeses in the United Kingdom (whether home-produced or imported) were contaminated.[25] It is obvious that 'open government' on public health matters had not been politically expedient until the degree of public alarm became a counter force to the influence of groups with a vested interest in profitable food production. The problem is a familiar one in health education, affecting accurate information about food safety, nutrition and diet, and effective warnings about the noxious effects of smoking and alcohol.

Thus the recent British excitement over eggs and soft cheese provides a cautionary tale for those with high ideals in health education. The United Kingdom is certainly not alone in its problems over food safety. A recent WHO survey[27] has shown that throughout Europe there is poorly coordinated control over safety of the production, storage, and marketing of food. In contrast, the US Food and Drug Administration has at its disposal wide powers of surveillance and control and can prosecute the producers of contaminated foodstuffs. There is little point in idealistic discussion of autonomy in health education if the legislation and the institutions do not exist to protect the consumer from concealment of unsavoury and economically embarrassing information. Autonomy for the recipients of health education can be ensured only if the educators are genuinely free from government interference, while being fully supported with funding and up-to-date information by the government. Any society which seeks to establish a genuine programme for health education must devise legislation which prevents indoctrination by those with either political or financial advantage to be gained. Unfortunately the trend in the United Kingdom has been towards an ever greater central control of information and the political independence of the health education bodies in both England and Scotland has been severely compromised. Thus, as the year 1992 approaches, perhaps a political objective for those concerned for the health of Europe should be political autonomy for health education in order to promote informed and autonomous choice by all those affected by the many health hazards of our affluent societies.

REFERENCES

 1. Illich, I. *Limits to Medicine*. London: Penguin, 1977.
 2. Kant, I. *Fundamental Principles of the Metaphysic of Morals*. Translated by K. Abbot. New York: Bobbs-Merrill, 1949.
 3. Downie, R.S. and Telfer E. *Respect for Persons*. London: Allen and Unwin, 1969.
 4. Harris, J. *The Value of Life*. London: Routledge and Kegan Paul, 1985.
 5. Lindley, R. *Autonomy*. London: Macmillan, 1986.
 6. Peters, R.S. (ed.). *The Concept of Education*. London: Routledge and Kegan Paul, 1967.
 7. Peters, R.S. Aims of education—a conceptual enquiry. In: R. S. Peters (ed.). *The Philosophy of Education*. Oxford: Oxford University Press, 1973.
 8. Langford, G. and O'Connor, D.J. (eds.). *New Essays in the Philosophy of Education*. London: Routledge and Kegan Paul, 1973.
 9. Quoted in Snook, I.A. (ed.). *Concepts of Indoctrination*. London: Routledge and Kegan Paul, 1972.
10. Thompson, I.E. Health education. In: Campbell, A.V. (ed.). *A Dictionary of Pastoral Care*. London: SPCK, 1987.
11. Draper, P., Griffiths, J., Dennis, J. and Popay, J. Three types of health education. *Br Med J* 1980; **281**: 493–495.
12. Coutts, L.C. and Hardy, L.K. *Teaching for Health*. Edinburgh: Churchill Livingstone, 1985.
13. Seedhouse, D. *Health: The Foundations for Achievement*. Chichester: Wiley, 1986.
14. Tones, B.K. *Effectiveness and Efficiency in Health Education: A Review of Theory and Practice*. p. 12. Edinburgh: Scottish Health Education Unit, 1977.
15. Baelz, P. Philosophy of health education. In: Sutherland, I. (ed.). *Health Education: Perspectives and Choices*. London: George Allan and Unwin, 1979.
16. Snook, I.A. *Indoctrination and Education*. London: Routledge and Kegan Paul, 1972.
17. Smart, P. The concept of indoctrination. In: Langford, E. and O'Connor, D.J. (eds.). *New Essays in the Philosophy of Education*. London: Routledge and Kegan Paul, 1973.
18. Wilson, J. Indoctrination and rationality. In: Snook, I.A. (ed.). *Concepts of Indoctrination*. London: Routledge and Kegan Paul, 1972.
19. Williams, G. Health promotion—caring concern or slick salesmanship? *J Med Ethics* 1984; **10**: 191–195.
20. *The Guardian* 2 March 1989.
21. Galbraith, N.S. Chicken and egg. *Br Med J* 1989; **297**: 704.
22. Editorial. *Salmonella enteritidis* phage type 4: chicken and egg. *Lancet* 1989; **8613**: 720–22.

23. Coyle E.F. *et al*. *Salmonella enteritidis* phage type 4 infection: association with hens' eggs. *Lancet* 1989; **8623**: 1295–1296.
24. Editorial. Salmonellosis and eggs. *Br Med J* 1989; **297**: 1557–1558.
25. Editorial. Anything to eat? *Lancet* 1989; **8635**: 416–418.
26. News. Safer eggs on the horizon. *Br Med J* 1989; **298**: 209.
27. World Health Organization. *Public Health in Europe 28. Food Safety Services*. Second edition. Copenhagen: WHO Regional Office for Europe, 1988.

CHAPTER 3

Health Education: The Ambiguity of the Medical Role

RAANAN GILLON

SUMMARY

In this chapter I address some of the ethical problems that confront doctors when they wish to act not only as therapeutic agents but also as health educators or promoters. Using the framework of four widely accepted moral principles—respect for autonomy, beneficence, non-maleficence, and justice—I conclude that health education is faced by the same sorts of moral tensions that arise in other aspects of medical care.

INTRODUCTION

Health education has been an aspect of enlightened medical thinking since Hippocratic times, at least in the general sense that such members of the medical profession have seen it as part of their job not merely to try to cure disease but also to try to prevent it and to promote better health.[1] Today, health promotion not only remains an integral part of medicine but doctors are being ever more urgently encouraged to practise it routinely,[2] and many other groups apart from doctors are involved, including a variety of health care professionals, health educators, and politicians. To judge from the almost messianic fervour of its enthusiasts, health education is an unmitigated good to be pursued eagerly and acceptingly. Those who criticize it tend to be relegated to the same class of fringe maverick as those who criticize motherhood. In this Chapter I wish to discuss some of the ethical problems that confront doctors when they wish to act not only as therapeutic doctors but also as health educators or promoters. Using as a framework for analysis four widely acceptable moral principles or values—respect for autonomy, beneficence, non-maleficence, and justice—I conclude that health education, far from being the unproblematic good that its enthusiasts so often depict, is in fact faced by the same

Ethics in Health Education
Edited by S. Doxiadis. ©1990 John Wiley & Sons Ltd

sorts of moral tensions that arise in other aspects of medical care, itself seen as a prima facie good which nonetheless confronts a variety of moral problems in its applications.

SOME EXAMPLES

Some examples may help to indicate the range of possible ethical worries arising out of health education in medical practice.

1. It is well known that even fairly 'normal' amounts of smoking, drinking (of alcohol), and eating (for example, of fats and sugar) are likely to damage people's health. How much should doctors try to influence, modify, or even override their patient's lifestyle preferences when such preferences are in the doctor's view unhealthy? Should they mark the notes or computer files to indicate the person's unhealthy tendency, and exercise health education whenever the patient attends the surgery, even for unrelated matters? Should the patient's permission be sought for such regular questioning and advice? What should the doctor's response be if such permission were refused, indeed if the patient told the doctor that such matters were none of his or her business? How justifiable would it be for doctors to withold medical care from patients who rejected their medical advice about how to prevent a particular illness—for example, to stop smoking? Consider both a general practitioner who refuses to treat a patient with antibiotics for an acute attack of bronchitis, when the chronic bronchitis leading to the attack is very likely to have been caused by heavy smoking, and a heart transplant surgeon who refuses to do a heart transplant on a patient because he has not given up smoking. How justifiable would it be for doctors to strike patients off their lists—that is, to refuse to treat them again—for not carrying out their health education advice?

2. A patient comes to the doctor about his ingrowing toenail. The doctor 'opportunistically' takes the patient's blood pressure. Before doing this, should he discuss the implications of finding raised blood pressure and ask whether or not the patient, on informed reflection, *wants* to risk a lifetime of blood pressure checks, worries, treatment side-effects, and even invalidism if the blood pressure is found to be raised?

3. Women who want the Pill for oral contraception are often routinely required to give a full medical history and undergo examination including vaginal examination and cervical smear and breast examination, often with instruction in self-examination for breast lumps. Lives are undoubtedly saved by such screening, but at the cost of considerable anxiety for many people, not only at the prospect of such intimate examinations but also after a possibly positive finding has been identified. A large percentage of such positive findings eventually prove negative but during their further investigation many people suffer great worry. Should doctors discuss the benefits and disadvantages of such screening before seeking their patient's consent to have it carried out?

4. Sometimes physical symptoms are diagnosed as resulting from stressful lifestyles. Doctors may then advise their patients to change their lifestyles— for instance to work less hard, be less ambitious, see more of their families and less of their offices. The evidence for a causal relationship between stressful lifestyle and medical problems may often be no better than speculative. How much should doctors advise people to change their lifestyles in such circumstances?

5. How much should doctors 'lean on' parents to have their infants immunized according to Government-advised schedules against common childhood illnesses, if the parents do not want the immunizations carried out?

6. How much should doctors 'lean on' pregnant women to change their unhealthy lifestyles if those lifestyles (notably heavy smoking and heavy alcohol drinking) threaten the health of the embryo/fetus/baby?

7. If patients want full health screening from their doctors, of the sort offered by private medical organizations at very considerable cost, because of the time and extensive testing required, should the doctors provide it?

8. If doctors wish to spread a particular health promotion message widely so as to benefit the public, should they use non-cognitive advertising techniques known to attract and persuade, such as the use of sexual symbolism?

My suspicion is that opinions within the medical profession as well as among the public would vary considerably and vigorously about the proper answers to these questions. In what follows I shall try to offer some medicomoral analysis applicable to such issues based on the four prima facie principles or values discussed by Beauchamp and Childress[3] and compatible with a wide variety of moral theories and perspectives. These principles are respect for people and their autonomy, beneficence, non-maleficence, and justice, with careful consideration of the scope of each principle an implicit requirement.

RESPECT FOR AUTONOMY

This prima facie principle requires people to respect the autonomy or self-deliberated self-determination of other people in so far as such respect is compatible with respect for the autonomy of all affected. In the context of health care, it requires health care workers not to impose but to offer their assistance, to do what they do only with the adequately informed consent of their patients or clients, to be honest and avoid deception, to keep their promises, and to respect their client's secrets and confidences. Like all four of these principles this is a prima facie principle and may have to give way to some other overriding moral concern. But in the absence of such overriding moral obligations, respect for patients' autonomy is required from doctors and other health care workers.

If such a principle is taken seriously it has important implications for health education. For the first question it raises in all the examples above, and in any other involving a sufficiently autonomous patient or other person, is: 'Does what

I propose to do respect the other person's autonomy?'. Now it can reasonably be inferred that when a patient consults a doctor about a particular problem he or she is doing so autonomously and expects the doctor to offer expert advice about how to resolve that problem. It does not necessarily follow that the patient will accept the advice, neither with justification can such acceptance be simply inferred. Thus in the first sort of case the doctor may well offer advice about the medical dangers of smoking, drinking, and overeating; but if the patient refuses that advice the doctor does not manifest respect for the patient's autonomy by berating the patient for failing to accept it, by going on repeating the advice (unless the patient indicates a readiness to accept such repetition), or by refusing to treat the patient's illness because the advice had not been followed. (The case of refusing a heart transplant to a patient who continues to smoke raises additional issues concerning both the probability of successful treatment if smoking continues and how best to distribute very limited and expensive resources, to which I return below.)

It might be argued that since respect for autonomy requires respect for the autonomy of all affected, the doctor's autonomy also requires respect and thus that he should be justified in requiring his patient to carry out his advice and in refusing to treat the patient unless he did. Certainly the doctor's autonomy is also worthy of respect just as anybody else's is, but two further issues arise. The first is that autonomy means *self*-rule (literally) and thus, although respect for people's autonomy requires respect for their self-rule, it does *not* require respect for their rule of others. One is not required to assist or allow people to do things to others against their wishes by the principle of respect for autonomy. Still, it might be argued, there is no reason for the doctor to go on treating a patient who rejects his advice. Respect for the doctor's autonomy should justify his withdrawal from the case and advice to the patient to try and find another more compatible doctor. So far as respect for autonomy is concerned this seems correct—a patient is not justified by this principle in demanding that a doctor does something which goes against that doctor's deliberated judgment. But whether the doctor still has some obligation to treat the patient, despite not being required to do so by the principle of respect for autonomy, remains an important moral question. However, the issue now turns on the second and third principles, beneficence and non-maleficence.

BENEFICENCE

Most moral theories incorporate *some* moral obligation to help *some* others. The scope and extent of this obligation, however, varies widely from theory to theory, and indeed disagreement about the scope and extent of beneficence may be seen as one of the main areas of dispute between different moral and political theories— whom do we have an obligation to benefit and how much of an obligation do we have to them? However, certain obligations are common to all theories and these include certain obligations of kin (for a reasonably uncontentious example consider the obligations of parents to their children) and obligations that have been positively and voluntarily undertaken. The obligations of friends to each other is perhaps the most obvious of these but doctors' obligations to their patients also seem to fall into the category of positively and voluntarily undertaken obligations of beneficence—for doctors positively and voluntarily join a profession whose members have undertaken to benefit their patients. There are of course many other groups who positively and voluntarily undertake obligations of beneficence to others. My favourite example is that of lifeboat men whose undertaking of beneficence is accepted at far greater risk of personal harm than arises in my own profession—and some claim that we *all* have *equal* obligations to benefit each other. My point here is that whether or not we accept the claim that people generally have an obligation to benefit each other, and regardless of disagreement about which groups accept obligations to benefit which other people, almost everyone accepts that doctors *do* have such an obligation to their patients, *at least* because they have voluntarily avowed such an obligation and it is accepted in most moral or political theories that people should stand by their voluntarily undertaken commitments. The extent of the *political* disagreement about how much of an obligation of beneficence we all have to each other is clearly discernible in contemporary British party political stances on this issue. Thatcherite conservatives have donned the mantle of nineteenth century laissez-faire liberals for whom beneficence to others, even the poor and needy in one's own community, is in general a morally optional activity, a matter of charity. The socialists, on the other hand, believe that benefiting others, especially the poor and needy, is not a moral option but morally obligatory, overriding respect for the autonomy of those who do not wish to undertake such beneficence. This position, in its starkest marxist form, is quite uncompromising in its imposition of the obligation of beneficence on others—'to each according to his need, from each according to his ability'.

Now if it is accepted that doctors have this obligation of beneficence to their patients then to that extent they restrict their own autonomy, notably their autonomy to refuse to benefit their patients. There is no reason for this to be an unlimited abnegation of autonomy, but doctors cannot, even if others can, simply withhold benefits from their patients, on the grounds that they do not wish to provide them to those who do not take sufficient notice of their advice. For they have taken on a general obligation to provide medical benefits to their patients, not merely those benefits that they chose to provide. The fact that a patient refuses the benefit the doctor thinks is most beneficial does not in itself prevent the doctor from offering some other benefit he may have at his disposal. Thus, although respect for the doctor's autonomy might justify the doctor's withdrawal of care in cases where patients refuse to carry out the preventative strategies they recommend, the obligations of beneficence that doctors autonomously choose to owe their patients may well negate such an unhelpful response. In the context of health education this is of obvious potential relevance to cases where doctors are inclined to withdraw their services if their patients refuse to take up the healthy lifestyles advocated by their doctors. The patient may go on smoking till he is (literally sometimes) blue in the face; still a doctor who takes seriously his self-imposed and professional obligation to benefit his patient ought to treat the patient if that is what the patient on reflection wants him to do, if some treatment is available which will provide net benefit to the patient, and provided that the treatment falls within the requirements of justice, of which more later. The same applies to other unhealthy lifestyle 'offences' which the doctor may believe his patient to commit. Of course, that in no way prevents the doctor from *advising* that the most effective way of regaining and maintaining health is to alter one's lifestyle in the relevant way. But coercion will generally be contraindicated by the requirement to respect people's autonomy, and withdrawal of care from those who reject one's advice will generally be contraindicated by a doctor's personally and professionally undertaken duty of care, or obligation of beneficence.

NON-MALEFICENCE

Whatever their stance over beneficence, all moral theories of which I am aware agree that each of us has a prima facie moral obligation to all other people to avoid acting so as to harm them. Thus even those theories that have little or no place for a universal obligation of beneficence nonetheless require a universal (though still prima facie) obligation of non-maleficence. Because of this, it is important I believe to keep these two principles conceptually separate. However, whenever one is attempting to exercise one's obligations of beneficence one inevitably risks harming the subject of one's attentions, and in medical practice this is peculiarly and increasingly true. Thus while one can contemplate the obligation of non-maleficence quite independently of any obligation one may or may not have of beneficence, it is always necessary when contemplating one's potentially beneficent actions to consider at the same time their potential for harm. This balancing of harms and benefits is a central concern of medical ethics, and in the sphere of treatment for illness well recognized. In the sphere of health education the recognition seems less widespread.

The obligation takes two distinct forms. On the one hand is a concern for the harms and benefits to everyone affected—the utilitarian central concern. I shall return to this general concern when considering obligations of justice. On the other hand, and the central preoccupation of those in the caring professions, is a concern for the harms and benefits to the individual patient. It is in this area that many of the moral problems of therapeutic medicine reassert themselves in relation to preventative medicine and health education. Thus, as with harm and benefit analysis in general, we need to identify the various harms and benefits anticipated from alternative courses of action and also at least an approximate assessment of the probability of each. As soon as we try to do this, in relation to the individual whom we propose to benefit by health education, the problems become apparent. How reliable is our evidence that self-palpation for breast lumps will actually improve the longevity of those who discover such lumps? What is the probability that any reliably established such benefit will occur for any individual woman who discovers such a lump? What about the correlative harms? Among these, as Williams points out, are the 'chore and tension' of regular self-examination.[4] For some women, as I can vouch from my own clinical experience, such tension can be very considerable. Then there are the considerable harms of discovering a breast lump—the anguish as it often is, of anticipating breast cancer, the hospital visits and investigations. There is too a distinct probability of being a 'false positive'—that is to say of having a benign breast lump.

The same sorts of potential harms, to weigh against the potential benefits, extend to any other screening programmes. In Chapter 4 of this volume Gorovitz points out that screening tests with even very high specificities and sensitivities—for example, 98% for each, in his instance—when applied to large populations having a low prevalence of the condition being screened for, can result in fairly low probabilities that those found positive actually have the condition. It must in fairness be added that the probabilities of false positives where there is a low prevalence of the condition searched for can be made to become extremely small. In a report on the false positive rates in an AIDS virus screening programme by US military,[5] for example, there was only one false positive in 135 187 persons tested. However, that still amounted to one false positive out of the 15 positives identified—that is, 6.7% of the positives identified were false positives. All such information can be important in weighing up the benefits and harms for the individual concerned.

In some cases there may not be any medical benefit to set against the harms. For example, it would seem at first sight that multiphasic medical screening should offer considerable medical benefits to those screened—a sort of MOT test for people to detect things going wrong before the person, like the car, breaks down. Yet a general practice prospective study in the 1970s showed clearly that when middle-aged people were randomly allocated into either a screening group or a conventional medical care only group, there were no significant differences in medical outcome between the two groups, despite the application of extensive health questionnaires and clinical tests to the screened group.[6]

Finally, there is the question of whose benefits and whose harms—a question of scope. For just as in medical research there may sometimes be a conflict between the doctor's primary duty to his patient and his duty to other patients including patients in the future, so in health education there may be similar conflicts, especially, as Skrabanek points out,[7,8] where the health education interventions are themselves being researched. Other problems of such conflicts arise in AIDS virus screening where the benefit is primarily for the public health but the harm may be great for those identified as positives.[9]

I am not of course to be construed as denying that net benefit over harm *can* be obtained from health education by the individual concerned. That would be absurd when so much evidence exists for the benefits of medical intervention to help people who wish to cut down their smoking (with correlated evidence of the dangers to health of smoking), who wish to improve their diet (with some reasonably reliable evidence that to do so will reduce the probability of ill-health), who wish to cut down their excessive alcohol consumption (with good evidence of the health risks of excessive alcohol consumption), and so on. But the evidence varies, and the probabilities both that certain sorts of screened for states cause ill-health and the evidence that changing such states prevents that ill-health also varies. In weighing up the harm–benefit ratio for the individual patient or client such information is crucial and often not available or not considered when deciding how vigorously to encourage patients to accept interventions to promote their health.

A further consideration in evaluating harms and benefits for the patient is that a person's own evaluation of harms may be quite different from that of his or her doctor. Thus, asking the patient is likely to be the best way of finding out whether, for example, a particular patient would find that knowing he or she had a raised blood pressure with the recommendation to attend to that blood pressure for the rest of his or her life, in the interests of reducing the risks of stroke and heart attacks was an acceptable harm to risk in the interests of possibly better health. Most people probably *would* wish to know their blood pressure, despite the risks of becoming to some extent made an invalid by discovering that it was high, but undoubtedly some would prefer not to know. Yet how many of us in general practice routinely explain such benefits and disadvantages before carrying out what is known as 'opportunistic' screening of our patients' blood pressures when they consult us for other reasons? I have to confess that my own explanation is a very limited one—something like 'while you are here would you like me to take your blood pressure?, assuming of course that you would wish to know you had raised blood pressure if by any chance you have'. Should I not be rather more informative, and offer counselling or at least a short written note about the benefits and disadvantages of having blood pressure taken? Yet the very idea seems slightly absurd so heavily socialized am I into the norms of medical practice.

WHAT IS THIS HEALTH?

So far I have been writing about the harms and benefits of preventing or reducing the chances of ill health, illness, or disease. But health promotion is potentially a far wider enterprise than the mere reduction of the probability of disease and that fact too raises important moral dilemmas in the context of harms and benefits. Perhaps the most important of these derives from the varied definitions of that 'health' which health education seeks to promote. According to typically medical definitions, health is the absence of illness or disease, and the proper role of doctors and health care workers is to try to treat and prevent such illness and disease. More ambitiously broad definitions of health see it not merely as the absence of disease but, in the words of the World Health Organization's (WHO) account of the matter, as a 'state of complete physical mental and social well-being'.[10] Now if *that* is to be the definition of health, and health promotion is to be the proper concern of doctors and other health care workers, one can begin to sympathize with the fear expressed by Carlyon that God has been turned into a doctor.[11] For few enterprises in a person's life are *not* concerned with either physical or mental or social well-being or some combination and thus few enterprises fail to become the legitimate concern of a doctor interested in promoting the WHO sort of health.

Do we as a society really *want* people like me to be legitimately concerned with promoting everybody's health in this immensely broad sense of the term? The answer may depend, among other things, on (a) whether we do so in an autonomy-respecting way, so that we offer rather than impose our interventions and on (b) whether we restrict ourselves to those very limited aspects of health education in which we can properly claim some skills. Let me explain. Another word for health in the WHO sense might be the ancient Greek word for human flourishing in its totality—*eudaimonia*. Health education then becomes no less than the promotion of eudaemonia or human flourishing. I would flourish if I could play good music, but I can't; you would flourish as a poet but you aren't very good at writing poetry; she would flourish if only she could run fast enough to join the team (or lift a heavy enough weight!) but she can't; he would flourish if only he could get a first-class degree, but he seems unlikely to do better than a lower second. All of us are manifesting inadequacies in our health, by manifesting less than *complete* physical, mental, and social well-being. Given the presuppositions noted above, we doctors should presumably be trying to remedy *all* these inadequacies. But are we any good at those sorts of health education? One has only to press at the implications of accepting this broad meaning of 'health' to conclude that at the very least we doctors should be extremely modest in claiming any skills in health education, if the WHO definition of health is accepted. The skills we have been trained in simply do not address the vast majority of ways in which people can attain WHO health or eudaemonia, and if we tried to help without such skills we almost certainly would fail. We *have* been trained to some extent in that narrow sector of health education that relates to prevention of disease and illness and thus to the promotion of eudaemonic health in so far as such prevention contributes to eudaemonia. We should be explicit about our limitations as doctors in being able to help people attain that perhaps ideal and certainly mythical state of *complete* physical, mental, and social well-being to which some may wish to aspire.

JUSTICE

The fourth prima facie moral principle or value that all moral theories incorporate is that of justice, some requirement for fair adjudication between competing claims, whether in the realm of distributing scarce resources, respecting people's rights, or following the requirements of morally acceptable laws. Moreover all theories of justice incorporate some requirement of equality of treatment, though—as Aristotle reasoned so clearly—the requisite equality of treatment has to be in relation to some other quality. Moral and political theoreticians have continued to argue ever since about what the relevant other qualities are—is it, for example, to be equal treatment in relation to equal need, or in relation to equal rights, or in relation to equal benefit, or to equal wealth, or to equal ability, or to equal contribution, or to equal past or future merit, or to what? Let me simply assert here that whatever one's overall theory of justice is to be, distribution of medical resources must include, as a *necessary* condition, distribution in relation to medical need (on pain of near incoherence—imagine distributing medical resources *without* regard to medical need). On the other hand, even if *all* available resources were to be distributed to medical care it still seems highly likely that not all medical need could be met by those resources. Thus the requirement for just distribution of inadequate medical resources would remain even in such implausible political cirmumstances, let alone in those that actually exist, with demand for resources for medical care having to compete with all the other reasonable demands for resources. In such a situation medical need, while affording a *necessary* condition for just distribution of medical resources, cannot be *sufficient*. Whatever additional criteria are to be accepted, some way of comparing the claims of the competing candidates for meeting medical need must clearly be found. This is an area of ethical analysis that has so far received inadequate attention, let alone successful resolution, but presumably whatever system is chosen, health education techniques will properly have to compete with all the other medical techniques available for improving people's health. Furthermore, it seems at least plausible to assume that whatever system for just allocation of scarce medical resources is chosen, cost per unit benefit will be one of the criteria, in addition to that of meeting medical need, to require consideration.

In that context health education projects may or may not prove to be the best choice when compared with merely therapeutic activities. For instance, although it is supposed to be a truism that 'prevention is better than cure', the 'better' may not be affordable—and, as Charny and Roberts[12] argue, worth is not the same as affordability. A striking example should make the point. The cost of saving a life through routine cervical cytology is assessed as somewhere in the region of £270 000–£285 000 (along with the concomitant need for 401 000 smears and 200 excision biopsies).[13] By contrast, the cost of saving one life by breast cancer screening using routine mammography between the ages of 50 and 65 years is calculated to be £39 000.[14] Compared with this, the cost of saving a life by appendicectomy for actue appendicitis, or of pneumonia by the use of antibiotics, is very cheap. So too, however, is the cost of saving a life by advice from the general practitioner to stop smoking. Once again the point of this analysis is not to show that preventative strategies are in general more expensive or otherwise worse than treatment strategies, but only to show that as with all other aspects of health care, prevention has to be assessed not only for its benefits but also for its costs, both to the recipients as indicated above, and also to the providers of the resources, which increasingly means taxpayers and insurance premium payers or both, and to those who are denied benefits as the result of such costs (opportunity costs, as the health economists call these).

Justice as respect for rights will also impinge on health education as it does on other areas of health care. According to an optimistic editorial in the journal *Health Promotion*, 'health is moving towards the status of a universal human right' and 'health policy should move beyond disease prevention to a positive promotive position'.[15] Apart from doubts about what it might *mean* for health to be 'a universal human right'—presumably the author means that some adequate degree of health *care* is 'moving towards the status of a universal human right'— the claim requires very careful analysis. How much health care (including health education and preventative health care) is to be 'a universal right' and against whom is the right to entail the reciprocal obligations (for every right entails a duty on someone, by definition)? What specific aspects of health education and preventative health care are to be considered as universal rights, and who have the corresponding duties to provide the necessary resources? These problems are addressed in a stimulating paper by Stacey?[16]

Another area of moral concern in the sphere of justice considered as respect for rights is the conflict between individual rights and public welfare. This is a common problem in the context of public health measures which impose health-related activities on all members of a given population for the general welfare—for example, immunization against infectious diseases or fluoridation of public supplies of drinking water. The health problems associated with smoking and alcohol have already been raised in the context of conflict between doctor and patient, but they arise again in the context of governed and government, when governmental action to forbid smoking and drinking, or even just to tax them prohibitively, are entertained. Do people have a right not to be interfered with by their governments for their own good? Is Bernard Levin right to rail that 'our world is overflowing with those who want to take away our pleasures, ostensibly on the ground that our pleasures are bad for us, though in fact because they cannot bear anyone enjoying anything anyway'?[17] Conversely, if people do not have the right to prevent their governments passing laws to stop them using heroin and marihuana then why should they have a right to stop them passing laws forbidding alcohol and tobacco? And finally, in the murky realm of rights, if people are to have a universal right to health care, can that right be overridden, as some advocate, if they have been the cause of their own ill-health by failing to live in whatever ways have been officially approved as 'healthy'?

It is in the context of moral issues such as those outlined above that the final component of justice—obedience to just laws—ought to be considered. For obedience to law is not necessarily morally obligatory (just think of your favourite properly breakable immoral law)—it is only morally acceptable laws that morally require to be obeyed. Of course what counts as a morally acceptable law when a community's moral views are divided about the issue in question is another unresolved moral question. But it is a question that is just as applicable to the arena of health education as it is to any other area of legislation.

CONCLUSION

In conclusion, then, health education is as heavily bedevilled by moral issues as is any other area of health care. Just as in recent times the moral issues arising in therapeutic medical care have been increasingly carefully identified and set against the enthusiasms of doctors and other health care workers for their potentially but not inevitably beneficial interventions, so too ought the moral issues of health education to be identified and set against the undoubtedly great potential benefits that this area of health care can also provide. In trying to achieve these objectives it seems reasonable to require health education to conform, as much as any other area of medical care, to the medicomoral norms of respect for people's autonomy, beneficence, non maleficence, and justice.

REFERENCES

1. Sigerist, H.E. *A History of Medicine*. New York, Oxford: Oxford University Press, 1961: 234–248.
2. Secretaries of State for Social Services, Wales, Northern Ireland and Scotland. *Promoting Better Health—The Government's Programme for Improving Primary Health Care*. London: Her Majesty's Stationery Office, 1987.
3. Beauchamp, T.L. and Childress, J.F. *Principles of Biomedical Ethics*. Second edition. Oxford, New York: Oxford University Press, 1983.
4. Williams, G. Health promotion—caring concern or slick salesmanship? *J Med Ethics* 1984; **10**: 191–195.
5. Burke, D.S., Brundage, J.F. Redfield, R.R. *et al*. Measurement of the false positive rate in a screening program for human immunodeficiency virus infections. *N Engl J Med* 1988; **319**: 961–964.
6. Holland, W.W., Creese, A.L. D'Souza, M.F. *et al*. (The South-East London screening study group). A controlled trial of multiphasic screening in middle-age: results of the South-East London screening study. *Int J Epidemiol* 1977; **6**: 357–363.
7. Skrabanek, P. The physician's responsibility to the patient. *Lancet* 1988; **i**: 1155–1157.
8. Skrabanek, P. Preventive medicine and morality. *Lancet* 1986; **i**: 143–144.
9. Blendon, R.J. and Donelan, K. Discrimination against people with AIDS—the public's perspective. *N Engl J Med* 1988; **319(15)**: 1022–1026.
10. World Health Organization. Basic documents: preamble to the constitution of the World Health Organisation. In Reiser, S.J., Dyck, A.J. and Curran, J.C. (eds.). *Ethics in Medicine*. Cambridge, Massachusetts and London: MIT Press, 1977: 552.
11. Carlyon, W.H. Reflections: disease prevention/health promotion—bridging the gap to wellness. *Health Values: Achieving High Level Wellness* 1984; **8(3)**: 27–30.
12. Charny, M.C. and Roberts, C.J. Public health and public wealth. The distinction between worth and affordability; implications of costs and benefits for the allocation of health care resources. *Postgrad Med J* 1986; **62**: 1107–1111.
13. Charny, M.C., Farrow, S.C. and Roberts, C.J. The cost of saving a life through cervical cytology screening: implications for health policy. *Health Policy* 1987; **7**: 345–359.

14. Knox, E.G. Evaluation of a proposed breast cancer screening regimen. *Br Med J* 1988; **297**: 650–654.
15. Draper, R. Healthy public policy: a new political challenge. *Health Promotion* 1988; **2**: 217–218.
16. Stacey, M. Strengthening communities. *Health Promotion* 1988; **2**: 317–321.
17. Levin B. Enter the tee-totalitarian. *The Times* 28 January 1988.

SECTION II

SOCIOPOLITICAL ISSUES

CHAPTER 4

Health Care Advertising: Communication or Confusion?

SAMUEL GOROVITZ

SUMMARY

Advertising of medical services of various sorts has been rapidly increasing, and now forms an important part of communication with the public about health care. There are many potential risks associated with such advertising, which can be motivated more by an interest in profit than in good public health. Some health care advertising is misleading, but strict regulation of advertising can be in conflict with freedom of expression and communication. It is prudent both to anticipate some of the ways in which health care advertising might damage the public interest and to consider modes of restraint that might make stringent regulation unnecessary.

INTRODUCTION

The issues discussed here concern economic pressures on health care institutions and the role of advertising as a response to those pressures as raised by recent developments in the United States. Despite great differences in the structure of health care between American and European countries, however, those issues have or are likely to have their counterparts in Europe. Growing forces in the direction of the privatization of health care will bring Europe some of the problems we now confront in the United States. For example, whereas physicians are now forbidden to advertise at all in the United Kingdom, if the government succeeds in making the provision of health care more akin to a market phenomenon, that could change abruptly. And, as several other chapters in this book make clear, questions of

Ethics in Health Education. Edited by S. Doxiadis. Published 1990 by John Wiley & Sons Ltd.
©1989 Samuel Gorovitz. This chapter is a revised excerpt from the author's book *Drawing the Line: The Thoughts of a Hospital Philosopher* to be published by Oxford University Press in 1990. It is based on experience as a Visiting Scholar in Residence at Boston's Beth Israel Hospital. An earlier version appeared in 1985 in the *Business and Professional Ethics Journal*.

the acceptability of medically related advertising are already raised in Europe in connection with such matters as the development of health education programmes aimed at children and the acceptance by various activities of promotional support from tobacco companies.

The significance of advertising in communication regarding health care will certainly continue to grow, and we will all face conflicts among the many financial interests that are increasingly interwoven with health care, our commitment to freedom of expression, our desire to protect the public against deception, and our sense of the mission of health care as a fundamental non-commercial commitment of any decent modern society. We are well advised to anticipate these issues and to think about them prospectively, before we have the need to resolve them.

The economic pressures on health care providers and institutions are rapidly growing more pervasive and visible throughout the developed world. Many factors, apart from inflation, contribute to this increasing presence of economic concerns in discussions about medical care. Some of these factors are traditional marketplace phenomena—for example, nurses, tired of being an underpaid profession, have sought wage increases that exceed the rate of inflation. In the United States, the price of liability protection has soared as a result of the increasing frequency of multi-million dollar judgments against health care providers in malpractice cases; the cost of these judgments and premiums significantly raises the price of health care services, as do the costs of medical tests that are done not because they are medically advised but because they strengthen the evidence—just in case it is needed—that the physician has been absolutely thorough. And medical progress itself contributes to the problem.

Although many medical advances make it less costly to treat a particular class of patients, some advances in health care increase the powers of medical intervention in ways that also increase costs. An example of the former is the development of the new immunosuppressive drug, cycolosporin A, which greatly increases the success rate for organ transplantation. Since it is far less costly to maintain a patient after a successful kidney transplant than to maintain that patient on renal dialysis, the availability of the drug is an advance that saves money.

Other advances, however, require immense expenditures. We need not look to exotic experimental devices like the artificial heart to find this effect. The computed tomography scanning equipment that became widely available in the 1970s required an investment of millions on the part of each hospital or medical unit that acquired it. Now magnetic resonance imaging devices offer a superior technology—sharper images without radiation risks—but this new equipment is even more costly.

Many couples who earlier would have had to live with their infertility, either remaining childless or else adopting children, now are patients in *in vitro* fertilization programmes sometimes costing tens of thousands of dollars. Victims who would have died at the scene of an accident or assault a few years ago are now rushed by helicopter to shock trauma units where their lives may be saved by extremely intensive care that is immensely expensive. New drugs, developed only after long and costly research programmes, require long and costly testing before they are approved for use as safe and effective; when they are finally on the market, they are priced to include the costs of research and testing, in addition to those of production, marketing, liability protection, and profit margin.

So the costs of medical care climb higher and higher, at a time of increasing pressure from various sources to contain them. In the United States, that pressure is not a reaction only to higher health care costs but is also due in part to such factors as concern with the weakness of the national economy that is reflected in an enormous federal deficit and our unfavourable international trading position.

To compete successfully with foreign manufacturers who have both highly efficient production technology and a very inexpensive labour force, American manufacturers must lower their production costs in every possible way. A major ingredient in the per-unit production costs of American manufactured goods—especially heavy goods such as motor cars and appliances—is the cost of health care insurance for employees. So employers want to contain or even reduce the cost of health care plans. The only ways to do that are to reduce coverage, to increase efficiency, and to reduce the actual costs of medical care. All these methods are being tried, but there is understandably great resistance to any reduction in coverage, especially as the costs of care are increasing. And only a limited amount can be achieved through increased efficiency. So limiting the costs of health care becomes a major focus.

At the federal level in the United States, there is some concern for that 15% of the American population who lack adequate access to decent medical care because of their poverty, but there has been even greater concern, at least within the Reagan administration, to reduce total federal expenditures for social programmes. Thus President Reagan, in his budget request for fiscal year 1987, tried to cut 70 billion dollars from federal outlays for health care.

The pressures that increase medical costs and the pressures to reduce them are thus on a collision course, with hospitals uncomfortably in the middle—most with decreasing occupancy rates that mean lower income in the face of rising costs. No wonder they are starting to think of the world of prospective patients as the marketplace; no wonder they are becoming more aggressively competitive with one another, no wonder that advertising has become a part of the marketing programme at many hospitals around the country.

'WE CAN'T WAIT TO GET YOU INTO OUR NEW OPERATING ROOM' *reads the headline of an advertisement by Virginia Beach General Hospital. The smaller print reveals that the hospital plans an open house to show the public its new surgical suites. I see a reprint of the ad in the latest issue of* Healthcare Advertising Review, *which describes the ad as 'calculated shock'. The review*

comments admiringly that 'The headline was, obviously, deliberately intended to shock people into a major bit of reading, even if it had to turn a few people off to do it. How well did it work? Over 800 people attended VBGH's open house ... and we really like the quality of the copy.'

Another headline catches my eye. 'ATTENTION MEDICARE PATIENTS' says the First Stop Medical Clinic of Racine, Wisconsin, and, below, 'This coupon is worth $100 toward a complete medical examination.' A discount coupon! The review's comment has a headline of its own, 'HARD SELL ... SELLS'. Indeed it does; I read that 'Ten to twenty new patients a day come walking into First Stop's 13 clinics, each holding a $100 coupon ... and each one a potential avenue to hundreds or thousands of dollars in Medicare and/or other third-party payments. A&P has been using this format to sell soup and soap and soda pop for years; now First Stop brings the "cents-off" coupon to patients in their Golden Years.'

Finally I get to the front of the magazine; I see that I can subscribe for $185 a year. The copy tells me why I should: 'Bring in the patients; bring in the profits! That's the undisguised goal of some of the finest advertising and promotion being done in America today ...' But I decide to do without its systematic collection of the best; I'll settle for what I come across on my own.

The rush toward aggressive health care marketing will surely continue, as the old restraints against advertising by professionals crumble away—much to the sadness of many doctors, lawyers, and hospital administrators whose sense of the dignity of their professions is assaulted by such developments. But their resistance is to little avail.

In Bates v. the Arizona Bar, the Supreme Court extended first amendment protection to advertising by attorneys.[1] The Bar Association of Arizona had argued against that extension, claiming that advertising by attorneys would have adverse effects on professionalism, would be inherently misleading, would promote groundless litigation, would increase costs, would lead to undesirable packaging of fixed price services, and would lead to extreme problems of enforcement. The Court found these claims to be without substance. But it held, importantly, that it is the duty of the Bar Association to ensure full disclosure in all legal advertising and to promote consumer education with respect to legal services. Further, the Court said that:

'Because of the complexity of legal services and the lack of public sophistication, higher standards of truth than those applicable to other forms of commercial speech might apply. In some situations, supplements to advertisements, such as of warnings or disclaimers, may be required to prevent deception. Finally, claims concerning the quality of legal services which cannot be verified may be prohibited as misleading.'[2]

More recently, the Virginia Code of Professional Responsibility was modified to allow attorneys to advertise without restriction, so long as the advertisements contain 'no false, fraudulent, or deceptive claim or statement.'[3] So an attorney in Virgina may advertise that she wins 97% of her cases, or that her settlements are on the average 17% larger than the norm for attorneys in the region with comparable types of practice, so long as such claims are not false, fraudulent, or deceptive.

Legal advertising is clearly on the rise and is now a part of the reality of professional competition. But health care advertising, a bit slower out of the starting gate, has now taken the lead in the area of professional services. Is this a problem? Need anything be done about it? We can approach these questions by considering what might be said in such advertisements, what it may be taken to mean, what dangers can arise, and what measures might be appropriate against such dangers.

More may well be necessary than reliance on the integrity of professionals, hospitals, the advertising agencies, and the media. We hear affirmations of integrity in all those quarters, but complacent reliance on them is unwise. Many—perhaps the vast majority—of profit-oriented executives are people of integrity who want to make money in a way that is honest and serves the public interest. Many copywriters will only write advertisements that are in good taste, and many newspapers will refuse to run ads that are deficient in any of a long list of respects. Most people are decent folks in most respects most of the time.

Still, some behaviour occurs nearer the edges of the statistical distribution. So we have laws against arson, looting, and assault, without suggesting that they are necessary to keep most people from behaving badly. And we have regulations to protect us against various kinds of malfeasance, not because we think they are likely, but because we know they are possible. We construct protections against damaging and deviant behaviour in various domains of activity, without indictment of those domains as a whole. Even if most advertising is admirable—a claim I would not want to have to defend—it is still wise to consider the possible pitfalls associated with unrestrained, irresponsible, professional advertising. This, I believe, is the perspective reflected in the Court's imposition of regulatory responsibilities on the Arizona Bar Association.

Physicians do not yet typically advertise as independent practitioners, but hospitals in America have become prominent advertisers of their services and facilities as the competition for patients increases, and health-related advertising is becoming more common in Europe. To facilitate speculation about where all this might lead, consider two hypothetical advertisements I wrote as heuristic examples a few months before arriving at Beth Israel Hospital—with no suggestion that any specific advertiser might use them. Imagine that they have appeared in your local newspaper.

The first one reads as follows:

****

An important notice from the Wholesome Hospital Corporation

SAFE!   EFFECTIVE!   SIMPLE!

Tired of tiny tots? Fed up with inconvenience and uncertainty?

Sign up now for our special

WEEKEND ESCAPE

All at one low package price, we will tie your tubes, and provide all related services including a deluxe room with color TV and telephone, and all meals. Transportation optional. Then, just three weeks later, at no extra charge...

Enjoy your new freedom at the nearby Eros Lodge Hotel with the guest of your choice, for two glorious days and one night, including continental breakfast for two and a welcoming bottle of champagne!

DON'T PROCRASTINATE; DON'T PROCREATE

Call our toll-free number now; major credit cards accepted.

800-101-0000

(Men! Ask about our Vasectomy Value Vacation)

Read these testimonials from satisfied clients!

Mrs. H.G. It was the best anniversary present Leo ever gave me.

Ms. W.N. I don't know why I waited so long. Your weekend special changed my life!

Mrs. R.V. I recommend you to all my friends. And to think the health insurance paid for it all! It's the best value around.

When it comes to your health, the Wholesome Hospital Corporation is always a step ahead!

****

I wrote that just to get into a copywriting frame of mind, and to get a sense of what might happen if hospital advertising became aggressive and unrestrained, even by canons of good taste. Of course no hospital would actually place such an advertisement. But it can be useful to have an example of what is clearly beyond the limits of appropriateness.

The second example is less obviously unrealistic:

****

An Important Message

to

HEART PATIENTS

from the

Wholesome Hospital Corporation

Last year hundreds of patients had elective heart surgery at Wholesome Hospital. Nearly all of them returned to good health. In fact, the mortality rate was just 2%. Hundreds of patients had heart surgery at Urban Central Hospital, too. But the mortality rate there was *300% higher*! In that teaching hospital, lots of young doctors and medical students are in training. At the Wholesome Hospital, only fully qualified surgeons are permitted to perform surgery.

The choice is yours.

When the time comes to schedule your bypass surgery, call us directly, or tell your doctor that you prefer Wholesome Hospital, the one with the high rate of success. And remember: When it comes to your health, the Wholesome Hospital Corporation is always a step ahead.

(Medicaid patients not accepted)

****

This advertisement, too, would distress me if it were actually placed by a hospital, despite the fact that (by hypothesis) there is no false claim within it. But it is not enough simply to judge an advertisement objectionable; the point is to clarify precisely just what about it is distressing. Knowing that may help us understand what limits, if any, should be placed on a hospital's freedom to advertise, or what limits to accept voluntarily about what one will or will not do in response to competition—and this is an issue that Boston's Beth Israel will surely have to confront.

To understand better how to get some endeavour right, it generally makes sense to look at examples of it going wrong, and to clarify what is wrong about them. One way to understand the ingredients of good medical practice is to examine specific instances of bad medical practice, identifying and analysing their deficiencies; the same approach can shed light on advertising practices in health care.

The advertisement for heart surgery is misleading in various ways, without resorting to falsehood. Studies of coronary arterial bypass surgery do indicate a range of mortality rates roughly from 2% to 6%. So Wholesome Hospital's (WH) mortality rate could well be 2%, while the rate at Urban Central (UC) could be 6%. But note that the rate given for WH is for elective surgery, while that given for UC is for all heart surgery. That difference alone could account for a difference in mortality rates.

The suggestion in the advertisement is that the difference in rates reflects a difference in quality of care, but it may reflect nothing more than a difference in the patient populations. This possibility is reinforced by the fact that WH declines to serve Medicaid patients, who are therefore likely to be a part of the UC population, and are also likely to be a population with poorer health and lower prospects of recovery. One very effective way of maintaining a high success rate is to refuse to take the very difficult cases, sending them instead to public hospitals which do not have the same luxury of turning them away.

Note also the suggestion implicit in the comment about staff responsibilities. True, UC is a teaching hospital. It is also true that at WH only fully qualified surgeons are permitted to perform surgery. One is invited to infer that at UC surgery is performed by the unqualified. But that is likely to be untrue. It may be that surgery is performed in part by surgeons in training under the supervision of more senior physicians, but it is not obvious either that they are therefore unqualified, or even that the standard of care is in any way lower than at UC. Indeed, it may even be that the combination of distinguished clinical faculty and surgeons-in-training, working under close scrutiny at WH, provides a higher level of skill overall than do the practitioners at UC.

Finally, note how the figures are presented. A mortality rate of 6% is obviously higher than one of 2%, although it is still fairly low. But the figure of 6% does not appear in the advertisement. Instead, we are told that the UC rate is '300% higher'— a dramatic difference indeed! The same statistics could be presented differently, of course. It could have been claimed that the success rate at UC is only 94%, while at WH it is 98%. That may be a significant difference, but putting the figures that way makes it plain that both hospitals have low mortality rates, and similar success rates. The advertisement is written to take advantage of the fact that statistical literacy is extremely rare and that these two different ways of representing the same data will have very different impact on typical readers. Thus, the reference to WH as 'The one with the high rate of success' reinforces the misimpression that UC has a low rate.

It is time to give my first seminar in the hospital. I gather my notes and papers, and head for the seminar room. About 40 people are there, a mix of doctors, nurses, students, health administrators, and miscellaneous tourists. I put them to work on an exercise designed to reveal how tenuous and unreliable our instincts about statistical matters tend to be. I ask them each to answer two questions on a handout sheet, and promise to report on their responses the next week. They have plenty of time; the sheet is passed out at the beginning of the seminar and won't be collected until the end.

Here is a slightly revised version of what the handout said:

Assume that the following information is true.

A new disease affecting people who read books about health care has recently been identified. It occurs in 0.1% of the population at risk. The symptoms are nasty, but the disease is not fatal. If it is left untreated, the victim has chills and fever for several weeks and suffers from moderate intermittent nausea and palsy. The symptoms then diminish and disappear. A new treatment eliminates these symptoms entirely, but it only works if administered before the onset of symptoms. That treatment involves no significant risk, and nearly always works. But it is costly, involves taking daily doses of a foul medicine, and, worse, requires total abstention from ice cream for eight weeks.

A new test has been developed to identify victims of the disease presymptomatically. Its specificity and sensitivity are each 98%; that is, it identifies 98% of those who have the disease with a positive test result, and it identifies 98% of those who do not have the disease with a negative test result.

The public health service has screened 100 000 potential victims of the disease with this test, in order to identify those who should be offered the treatment.

I regret to inform you that your test was positive. Please answer these two questions.

1. How likely do you think it is that you have the disease?

Probability: (check one) 95%+____, 85–94%____, 74–84%____, 65–74%____, 55–64%____, 45–54%____, 35–44%____, 25–34%____, 15–24%____, 5–14%____, 1–5%____, 0%____.

2. Do you want the treatment?

Take a few moments now to answer these questions for yourself. You need not calculate the answer to (1), just estimate what seems most reasonable. And you need not justify your answer to (2). I'll tell you in a few pages how the hospital staff answered, and how to think correctly about these questions. In the meantime, let's return to consideration of the advertisement by Wholesome Hospital.

This advertisement is misleading, so it would clearly be prohibited by any standard that effectively prohibits misleading claims. Would it be barred by regulations like that governing legal advertising in Virginia, which merely forbids 'false, fraudulent, or deceptive' claims or statements? The advertisement contains no false claims, so the question turns on whether it is fraudulent or deceptive overall. That will depend upon how strictly the notions of fraud, deceit and the misleading are interpreted, as well as on the effectiveness of monitoring and enforcement. A very strict interpretation might be hard to sustain, given the abundance of misleading advertising that surrounds us.

The advertisement is hypothetical, but the competitive phenomenon it reflects is not. The incursion of private for-profit hospitals into the market in competition with public hospitals has already resulted in fierce competition, with private hospitals sometimes skimming off the more profitable cases, leaving the public hospitals with a greater proportion of patients whose prospects of recovery are least or who cannot cover the costs of their care. The impact of the Wholesome Hospitals thus functions, at least in part, contrary to the public interest, though perhaps profitably for their stockholders.

The development of the for-profit hospital sector is very much a part of the health care scene in many regions. Even without it, some hospitals have already begun to advertise for patients. Such competition has prompted very aggressive advertising campaigns.

An article in *The Miami News*, under the headline 'Hospitals vie for patients with Madison Avenue flair,' reported in 1984 that 10 major hospitals in the area were spending $100 000 to $400 000 on annual advertising budgets—roughly 20 times what was spent just three years earlier.[4] Most of the advertising is positive in tone, simply emphasizing the virtues of what the hospitals provide. But the article quotes Ken Magee of the Florida Hospital Association as saying, 'We really are in a competitive marketplace right now... I think you will start to see some cutthroat competition, the kind that goes on in almost every marketplace.'

Back in my office, I tally the responses to my two questions about the hypothetical disease. Doctors and nurses, about two-thirds of the audience, were present in equal numbers—14 of each. Most of the doctors (over 60% of them) indicate that the likelihood of their having the disease, given the positive test result, is at least 95%. All but one of them judges the likelihood to be at least 85%. That one deviant respondent thinks it no more than 5%!

The nurses' views are more dispersed. Only 57% of them say the odds are at least 85%, and there are two maverick nurses who vote with the one dissenting doctor. The leftovers—neither doctor nor nurse—react somewhat differently. One-third of them (probably not a statistically significant number) say that the odds are not over 5%.

I notice a high correlation between answers to the first question and answers to the second one. The more likely a person thinks it is that he or she has the disease, the more likely it is that he or she has chosen the treatment. But there are exceptions; some of those who think the probability high nonetheless decline the treatment.

What the probability actually is can be calculated; it is a matter of demonstrable fact, not open to dispute. How a person responds to a treatment option is a different sort of matter; it just is not possible to get the second question demonstrably wrong. It is one of those value questions about a medical decision that is based on the relevant facts, but not capable of being derived from them.

Here, the factual and value aspects are separated into questions 1 and 2. No one seems confused about the difference between them; no one suggests that if the probability is high, it is a fact that treatment should be accepted. In the real world of medical care, facts and values swirl around together. It is easy to get them confused, and judgments about values are often disguised as statements of fact.

These figures do not surprise me. Sound statistical judgment is exceedingly rare, and I have used the exercise to make that point vividly to the Beth Israel staff. At the same time, I realize that it would have been comforting to find that these health care professionals are an exception.

I have promised to tell them next week about the exercise. It would be a great embarrassment to get it wrong myself when I tell them that most of them got it wrong. So I decide to run through the figures one more time:

The incidence of the disease is one-tenth of 1% of the population. So of the 100 000 people who have been screened, 100 (approximately) have the disease. The test identifies 98% of the disease victims with a positive test result, so it will product 98 positives—true positives—from those 100 people. The remaining 99 900 screened people do not have the disease, and the test will show that fact by providing most of them (98% of them) with a negative test result—a true negative.

But the test is not quite perfect; it will fail to identify 2% of those who are disease-free as being disease-free. It will give them a positive result—a false-positive—even though they do not have the disease. Since there are 99 900 without the disease, that 2% rate of false-positives will yield 1998 more positive results, all of them false. The total number of positives based on the screening of 100 000 people will therefore be 1998 plus 98, or 2096. But of these 2096 positives, only 98—4.7% of them—will be true-positives! So on the basis of the data provided in the statement of the problem, the likelihood of a person in the population at risk actually having the disease, given a positive screening test result, is less than 5%.

'Bravo!' for the deviant doctor and the two maverick nurses. I will go through the calculations at the next seminar, emphasizing that the point is not to embarrass anyone, but to underscore how pervasively devoid of even elementary statistical sense most people, including health care professionals, are. Medical education does not produce statistical literacy, even though medical decisions are largely based on statistics.

Consider now an actual advertisement placed by a medical centre in *The Miami Herald*. The advertisement invites readers to free cancer screenings, claiming that 'Last year we identified 427 suspected cancers after screening more than 2000 people.'[5] How are we to interpret such a claim? Grant that it is good for free screenings to be available and for people to take advantage of them. Consider what this advertisement says. The initial impact is that over 20% of those screened have suspected cancer—if we assume that 'more than 2000' stands for some number very close to 2000. If the actual number of people screened is much larger, the inference to a percentage will be proportionally erroneous. But even if the actual number is 2001, the impression given may be very misleading. For the advertisement says nothing about the screening technique used, so we have no information about its accuracy.

Assume that the actual rate of disease in the screened population is 3%. Then, of the 2000 subjects, 60 will have some relevant form of cancer. Assume further that the screening technique has a 98% sensitivity—that is, that it accurately identifies 98% of those who are afflicted. The process will then have identified 59 of the 60 cancer victims with positive test results. Add just one further assumption—that the screening technique has achieved its high sensitivity at the cost of achieving only a modest selectivity; it correctly yields a negative test result for 81% of those who are disease-free. Then, of the 1940 healthy individuals screened, 19%, or 368, will also have positive test results, although they will be false-positives. The total number of positive tests will thus be 427, as advertised. But of those 427 who are identified as suspected cancers, only 59—14%—will actually be ill. The other 86% of those who tested positive—368 people—will presumably go through some considerable terror before subsequently being confirmed as false-positives, and perhaps some of them will even be subjected to costly or harmful treatments for a disease they do not have.

It may well be worth subjecting them to that distress and risk in order to identify and help the 59 people who are diseased. Still, in deciding whether to present oneself for such screening, one might reasonably want to know about the incidence of the disease, the accuracy of the screening technique, and the availability of reliable methods of confirmation of initial test results. Perhaps the actual technique that was used is vastly better than what I have assumed here for illustrative analysis. But there is no way to know that from the advertisement.

The medical centre placing the advertisement has dual motivation. It wants to contribute to good health by identifying people who need treatment. But it also very much wants to be the provider of that and other treatments. So the screening programme also serves as a way of building connections with the community and of increasing the centre's visibility. Thus, the advertisement also says, 'Discover the New North Shore Medical Centre.' That is an entirely reasonable objective, but it conflicts with the disclosure of information about the screening programme that might decrease the reader's inclination to go to the centre to participate in the programme.

I do not condemn this advertisement in particular; I am concerned about hospital advertisements in general. Success rates are statistical information which is widely and notoriously misunderstood. The overall impression given by an advertisement containing statistical information may vary greatly from its literal content. This is so for two different reasons. First, there is the fallibility of the judgments people make about statistical matters, even when they are being deliberate and reflective.

This problem is well documented; contemporary cognitive psychologists have shown that people typically process statistical information in deeply flawed ways. There is an almost universal tendency to ignore statistically valid base-rate data, even when it is readily available, in the face of atypical, but vivid, anecdotal evidence or powerful visual images. (In the exercise I used, are people misled by the habit of thinking that 98% is typically an A+, so the test must be very good?)

This is a humbling fact about how the human mind works, but a fact nonetheless. If what is deceptive is that which induces, and can be reasonably expected to induce, beliefs that are untrue, then the perils of any essentially statistical advertising may be substantial.[6]

Second, and perhaps more important, is that advertising in any event is largely a non-cognitive interaction between advertiser and consumer. For that reason, it is a mistake to focus too narrowly on the cognitive content of advertising, looking only at the truth of its claims and the validity of its inferences. They may be no more than peripheral to how advertising works. There is a significant cognitive component in much advertising, sometimes conveying valuable information. But the reality of contemporary advertising is that the provision of accurate information to the consumer is often secondary or even absent; paradigmatic of such an information-free advertisement is one showing an attractive and apparently wholesome person in a beautiful setting smoking a cigarette, with the brand name of the cigarette the only verbal content of the advertisement.

Many advertisements avoid saying anything false by avoiding the assertion of any propositions whatever. This can be done by limiting the advertisement to visual images; it can also be done, after the fashion of some political speechwriting, by limiting the verbal content to the meaningless. An example of that is an airline advertisement some years ago affirming that 'Being first isn't everything, it's the only thing.' Or, perhaps it was 'Being first isn't the only thing, it's everything.' Since neither claim means anything, I cannot now remember which was the one in the advertisement. Such claims cannot be false because, lacking cognitive content, they cannot be either true or false. But they may play a role in deception, for the routes to deception are not solely cognitive. Our beliefs are determined only in part by rational judgment, just as our decisions are determined only in part by our beliefs.

Should we now regulate health care advertising, beyond the constraints which are imposed by current barriers to fraud and deception? Any response to this question will presuppose deep commitments about political theory and the proper role of government in relation to the public interest. Government must protect the public interest in various ways through regulation, but the stringency of regulations ought to reflect the degree of risk and the modes of redress that are available, and should not merely reflect the degree to which the behaviour in question offends the sensibilities of some people. Not everything deplorable ought to be regulated or prohibited.

Note also the considerable difference between goods and services. Goods are durable in time; even if the complaint is that they have broken or worn out prematurely, what remains can be examined long after the moment of acquisition. Further, manufactured goods admit of sampling techniques that can enhance quality control. Even so, it is often very difficult to obtain redress when one has been victimized by shoddy goods or deceptive advertising in relation to consumer goods. As Lee Weiner said, writing of the Federal Trade Commission's advertisement substantiation programme:

'An individual consumer's injury from deceptive advertising is typically too minor, in economic terms, to justify recourse to the judicial system ... even when consumers are aware that they have been victimized by fraudulent ad representations, little practical recourse is available.'[7]

Weiner goes on to argue that the FTC's effort 'to combat deceptive advertisements by eliminating representations that take advantage of the consumer's lack of technical expertise... has failed, on almost all counts, to achieve its goals.' Yet Weiner was writing of goods, with respect to which substantiation is considerably easier than with professional services.

Who might the victims be of deceptive advertising of health care services? We must know that before we can consider what modes of constraint might be appropriate. The most obvious victim is the direct consumer of misrepresented services. Competitors who lose business to the deceptive advertiser also are victimized. But there can be less obvious victims, as well. Identifiable persons depicted in an advertisement can be victims. This could be so, for example, if the facilities of a hospital's psychiatric unit were shown with a recognizable patient inadvertently visible in the background. More commonly, categories of persons exemplified by the individuals in an advertisement can be victimized; this has surely been the case with many advertisements depicting women and minority group members in ways that reinforce stereotypical images detrimental to their interests. Women are still the victims of much television advertising that continues to portray them in belittling, demeaning, and humiliating ways. Indeed, children and men are also victimized by such distorted images of women's roles. This victimization is a broadly based social phenomenon, far removed from the level of the direct consumer. In this respect, consider also car advertisements which have returned to an emphasis on speed, power, and 'macho' driving; the results may be—although this would be hard to document—an increased level of carnage on the highways and a corresponding increase in health insurance costs generally.

A profession, too, may be victimized by the advertising of one of its members, if that advertising misrepresents the nature of the profession or causes public opprobrium that is generalized, beyond the individual advertiser, to the image of the profession overall. So doctors and lawyers are properly concerned about advertising that might 'give the profession a bad name,' and hospitals are rightly concerned about the prospect of becoming involved in competitive advertising campaigns that diminish public respect for hospitals as institutions serving the public interest.

But at what level of generality is victimization by advertising the proper object of intervention—that of the direct consumer only, the broader social environment, or something between? This is a question of some complexity; the answer may depend on variable factors such as the level of risk and the available remedies for harms in each kind of circumstance.

To protect against victimizations of all these sorts, diverse constraints, beyond reliance on the good judgment of sponsors, already limit the content of advertising to some extent. A contemplated advertisement may be rejected because it violates the law, a code, or standard of the sponsoring industry or profession, the standards of the advertising agency, or the requirements of the media through which the advertisement is to be placed. Advertisements can violate none of these things, however, and still violate standards of taste. Each of these levels of restraint constitutes a protection against violations of certain sorts on behalf of potential victims.

A profession, through its own code of advertising standards, may be centrally concerned with protecting the reputation of that profession, and may forbid advertisements that would be inoffensive to a newspaper. But the newspaper, concerned with the social consequences of the stereotyping reflected in its advertisements, might in turn reject an advertisement that was not seen as offensive by the professional association.

This is as it should be. The various categories of potential victims of poor advertising constitute interest groups with different, although overlapping, concerns. Those interests are properly protected by different mechanisms, depending on the scope and severity of the harms at issue.

What restraints are needed on the advertising of health care services must be determined piecemeal, along with the development of such advertising. It may be that individual physicians, for example, possibly restrained by guidelines within their profession, will limit their promotional activity to a forthright and honest presentation of relevant information. Or it may be that the growing competition for health care resources, even in countries with national health insurance systems, will lead to aggressive and unrestrained promotion that will invite new mechanisms of constraint.

An advertisement for a physician in New York inquires, 'Psoriasis Sufferers, Why Suffer? 88% cleared!' Reprinted in *Hospital Tribune*, it illustrates a point emphasized by the article it accompanies—that medical advertising is on the rise, and will have to be taken into account even by physicians and hospitals hostile to advertising.[8] An adjacent article describes a physician in Milwaukee who budgets $100 000 a year to advertise the services of his four-person clinic, and whose aggressive marketing approach has prompted other physicians to advocate regulation by the profession that would place rigid controls on the content and form of medical advertising. That seems unlikely, in the judgment of an advertising agency professional who specializes in medical accounts, however; he told the newspaper that 'The Supreme Court has made it clear that so long as ads are not misleading or fraudulent or do not violate good taste, there is no limit on the content or medium.'

Will we see advertisement one day by the Wholesome Hospital? It is too soon to tell. Advertising by the major hospital corporations thus far seems tasteful and restrained. For example, the Hospital Corporation of America took a full page in the October 1984 *Smithsonian* to tell the story of how its newly acquired Navarro Regional Hospital was able to provide care to indigent and uninsured patients because of the innovative establishment of a Health Services Foundation, with funds from the sale of the hospital to HCA, in order to underwrite the costs of care for those not otherwise able to pay their bills. But HCA now controls over 400 hospitals. As it travels around the country—a corporate Pac-man gobbling up little hospitals by the day—in competition with Humana, other for-profit corporations, and the non-profit sector, will all the competitive gloves stay on? We may yet see advertising that is not demonstrably deceptive by legal standards, yet invites misunderstanding, serving the interests of the competing corporations in a manner that is contrary to the public interest.

I am not convinced that this will occur, but it would be naive to assume that self-restraint, good taste, and dedication to the public good on the part of corporate medicine and individual practitioners will prevent it. It may not be easy to decide what measures, of what degree of severity, will be appropriate to protect the public interest in respect to advertising of hospital services. But considering these matters prospectively may reduce the need for more stringent action later.

REFERENCES

1. Bates v. State Bar of Arizona, 433 U.S. 350, 1977.
2. Murdock, G.W. and Linenberger, P. Legal advertising and solicitation. *Land and Water Law Review*, 1981; V.XVI: 634.
3. *Virginia Code of Professional Responsibility*, D.R. 2-101, 2-102, 2-103, as quoted in Murdock and Linenberger, *op. cit.*, p. 648.
4. Papiernik, R.L. *The Miami News*. p. 16. 9 April, 1984.
5. *The Miami Herald*. 10 April 1984.
6. See, for example, *Judgment under Uncertainty: Heuristics and Biases*. Kahneman, D., Slovic, P. and Tversky, A. (eds.). Cambridge: Cambridge University Press, 1982,

especially Slovic, P., Fischoff, B. and Lichtenstein, S. Acts versus fears: understanding perceived risks. pp. 463–489.
7. Weiner, L.M. The substantiation program: you can fool all of the people some of the time and some of the people all of the time, but can you fool the FTC? *Am Univ Law Rev* 1981; **30–415**: 431.
8. *Hosp Trib* p. 20. 16 May 1984.

CHAPTER 5

Health Education: The Political Tensions

STEPHEN PATTISON AND DAVID PLAYER

SUMMARY

Health education is an activity undertaken amid considerable political pressures and it has substantial sociopolitical implications. In this chapter we explore some of the political tensions with particular reference to the work of the Health Education Council (1968–1987). After an initial discussion of relevant ethical factors and topics, two case studies are used to show what political pressures operate on health education in its constitution and practice. We conclude that state-sponsored health education occupies an ambiguous and circumscribed position in trying to promote comprehensive health in the entire population of the nation, but that this is not necessarily a reason for its not attempting to do so.

INTRODUCTION

In abstract and in general, everyone is against disease and illness and in favour of health. As soon as this ideal concept is given a specific content and meaning, however, it becomes controversial.[1,2] When it comes to the practicalities of working for health in a particular society, real conflicts start to rage. For any fleshing out of a vague ideal in reality precipitates antagonisms over definitions, values, means, and ends. If there are implications of change, there are bound to be individuals and groups whose vested interests, preferred habits, or cherished ideals are challenged. The fact of the matter is that health, health promotion, and health education are situated in a thoroughly political context. That is to say that health education is affected by and influences the

'activities of cooperation and conflict, within and between societies, whereby the human species goes about obtaining, using, producing and distributing resources in the course of the production and reproduction of its social and biological life.'[3]

Ethics in Health Education
Edited by S. Doxiadis. ©1990 John Wiley & Sons Ltd

In this chapter, the political context and tensions confronting one particular organization, the Health Education Council (HEC) for England, Wales and Northern Ireland, are used as case study material. One of the authors (DP) was Director General of the HEC from 1982 until its sudden and unexpected demise in 1987. His experience provides a unique resource for understanding the real political difficulties confronting such an organization in terms of its relationships with government and powerful social interest groups, such as the alcohol and tobacco industries. Political factors (understood in the broadest sense outlined in the definition above) impinge on all aspects of health education and promotion. This is clearly exemplified in a study of health information disseminated in a particular campaign on heart disease undertaken by the HEC, the findings of which are also outlined as a case study.[4]

ETHICAL ISSUES AND CONSIDERATIONS

Before moving on to the case study material, it will be helpful to abstract and note some of the ethical issues which arise in considering some of the political tensions surrounding health education.

Definitions

Defining is a highly political human activity undertaken by particular individuals and groups with a view to promoting some states or activities as against others. For this reason, the definition of terms like 'health education' and 'health promotion' is crucial as it will determine to a large extent what activities are included or proscribed. Inevitably, there are resource implications here. A government may well wish to fund health education understood as activity aimed at encouraging people to change their behaviour in a healthy fashion. It may baulk, however, at health promotion understood as doing whatever has to be done to improve the health of the population which might include political, legal, or fiscal action and education as well as information dissemination. It is important to identify the content, source, originators, and proponents of definitions if their practical and political implications are to be accurately assessed.

Responsibility

Responsibility is often alluded to in clinical medical ethics, but it is equally applicable to the sphere of health education, and in two main ways. First, it must be asked to whom health educators are responsible. Are they primarily responsible to their employers (mainly health or governmental authorities in the United Kingdom), or do they owe their main loyalty to the public at large, to particular groups, or even to specific individuals? There may be real conflicts of interest here; what is good for the public authorities may not necessarily be the best thing for members of the public themselves. Secondly, it may be asked who is primarily responsible for health and the elimination of illness in society. Much health education has tended to promote the idea that individuals are themselves the guardians of their own well-being. However, it is clear that major social forces impinge upon health. There are some forces affecting health upon which a government can act while an individual is relatively powerless—for example, environmental pollution. Who or what is responsible for health, in what circumstances, and to what extent?

Individual and Community

The modern ethical tradition in the West has tended to emphasize the centrality of individual autonomy and choice based on rational analysis.[5] Ethics has been blind to issues of corporate choice and destiny in a society where individualism is exalted as a supreme value.[6] Clearly, health education must wrestle with the tension between changing communities or even societies and changing individuals.[7]

Professions and Professionalism

Health education is regarded as a skilled activity which is undertaken by professionals. Some are medically or educationally qualified, others are qualified health educators. Whatever their route into health education, the fact that they see themselves as professionals poses problems of power, responsibility, and knowledge. Generally speaking, professions in Western society are powerful, conservative, relatively autonomous groups. Their training and codes of practice ensure high status and therefore draw members from the upper classes.[8–10] The question must then be asked to what extent do such groups share the interests and perceptions of the objects of their professional concern? Professionals are accorded much officially sanctioned power but their own interests and concerns may be divorced from those of the populace in general. They are not elected to their posts, nor, for the most part, do their professions come into existence by popular request. To what extent, then, do professional health educators have a right to change others? Do they really know best? By the same token, do not other members of society have a right to have their perceptions of health and illness taken seriously rather than having their knowledge and beliefs dismissed as 'folk tales'?[11–13] In attaining power and influence in society, professionals have tended to be individualistic in their approach to 'clients' in keeping with the dominant ethos of the West. It may be that this narrow focus should be challenged critically, for often the well-being of clients as individuals goes beyond individualized solutions. Neglect of the sociopolitical context will ensure that professionals fail in their stated aspiration to take the interests of those they serve as their own.[14]

Scope

It tends to be assumed that health education should be primarily addressed to those individuals who are likely to become ill.[15] It is they whose attitudes and behaviour patterns need to change. Yet, if the social and political factors in ill-health are clearly identified, it may be argued that it is health antagonists—for example, commercial companies, corporate bodies—who should be the primary objects of health education. It is their attitudes and activities which most need to be altered. The scope of health education is thus a very important aspect of considering political tensions and pressures.

Ends, Means, and Methods

Implicit in many of the former points are questions about ends, means, and methods in health education. The objectives identified for health education are arrived at through a broadly political process, but the means and methods used in this activity are also value laden. So, for example, an approach which emphasizes the importance of individuals' responsibility for their health buttresses the sociopolitical value of individualism over communitarianism. To emphasize the value of choice is congruent with the value of consumerism. Specific methods used, such as inviting people to read leaflets on their own as opposed to meeting in, say, self-help groups to develop communal understandings of what makes people ill and what would help to guarantee their corporate well-being, similarly carry a political message. Thus the methods used in health education can either reinforce or vitiate the ends sought. The medium is at least as important as the message, and has substantial ethical and political implications.

Justice, Equality, and Inequality

Situated centrally within society, it is impossible for health education to avoid issues of justice, equality, and inequality which affect the incidence of ill-health and the effectiveness and appropriateness of health education.[16-21] Health educators have to orient themselves within the ongoing debate on these issues, remaining clear that their work will affirm or challenge various perspectives implicitly or explicitly. There is no neutral stance. Every stance will help to support or question certain assumptions. They also have to decide whether they have an obligation to challenge what may be perceived as injustices and inequalities in their educational work.

Freedom

The values of freedom and choice are central to the Western democratic system. There is, however, considerable debate over the content of these values.[22] Individualist thinkers see freedom as minimizing constraint upon individuals; only when one person's freedom interferes with that of another should there be any intervention by the state or outside bodies, and then such intervention should be that of restraint until normal rights have been restored. At the other end of the political spectrum, collectivist thinkers argue that liberty is not simply a matter of freeing people from constraints; it is also necessary to equip and enable them to actually be and do things which are desirable. Broadly, this is the distinction between freedom as minimally and negatively defined as freedom *from* and freedom *for*, a more positive and potentially interventionist concept which implies the possibility of the state interfering in economies and the lives of people to enhance them and equalize liberty. In general, the political climate in Britain over the last decade or so has favoured the libertarian, individualist approach to freedom. Health education has, therefore, assumed that all members of society have equal choice and has sought to persuade and encourage them to make 'healthy' choices without state intervention. This has been accompanied by an unwillingness on the part of the state to intervene to make choices more possible. Thus, women are bidden to provide good food for their families by health educators, but government has felt it inappropriate to provide the social welfare benefits such as higher income support grants or free school meals which would help to ensure that good food is eaten.[23] At the same time, of course, the promotion of the notion of the freedom from restraint of the individual consumer maximizes the freedom of powerful interest groups such as the food industry to make financial gain from the populace by the unfettered marketing of their products.

Information and Truth

The truth about any situation—for example, why particular individuals or groups contract certain illnesses—is rarely clear and seldom simple. Reality is complex and there are usually a variety of causal factors involved.[24] This poses real practical problems for health educators, for they have to present a clear message, while knowing that it is only a partial message. So, for example, it may be desirable that people should stop eating certain kinds of foods for the good of their cardiovascular system. This is a clear message to put across, but it may also be true that social class position, poor living conditions, and stress contribute to heart disease. The problem then is how much should the public be told, how complex should the information which they receive be, and which aspects of causation and reality should be presented to them? Unedited presentation of all the 'facts' is less than useless in terms of getting a message across (unless the message is that there is no clear message, which might be the most honest response!). However, the need to arrive at simplicity and clarity can lead to biased and distorted views of the nature of reality and open health education to the charge of indoctrination. This is particularly true if information and messages seem to strongly confirm particular social values acceptable to those with great social and political power, rather than challenging those values. Once again, the individualization of explanations of illness, responsibility, and prevention might serve as a good example of this kind of bias. These issues border on the consideration of health education as ideology.[25] There are several ways of understanding 'ideology'. Perhaps the most common relates to using ideas and concepts to disguise and distort the nature of reality rather than to describe it accurately. Health education may be described as ideology in this sense when it distracts attention from primary causes and factors in causing ill-health—for example, environmental or social factors—to reinforce ideas that illness has only to do with individual attitudes and types of behaviour.

Interests

To be involved in education and change in society is to be situated amid the conflicting values, desires, powers, and struggles of many competing interest groups. Sometimes interests may be strongly and overtly expressed. So, for example, alcohol and tobacco companies openly want to encourage people to consume their products and so wish to minimize effective health education opposed to this. More covertly, sweet manufacturers or others may attempt to identify themselves with a drive towards effective health education by sponsoring activities which link their names with healthy activities. At another level, governments or other groups may claim in public that they wish to promote health but their actions may belie this claim and work against health educational aims, by underfunding them or by refusing to implement policies which would complement them while supporting policies which flatly contradict them. It must not be forgotten that ordinary members of the public also have health interests and needs which may be unarticulated, inadequately articulated, pluriform, covert, or overt. Just because ordinary people do not lobby hard and effectively for their own views and beliefs does not mean that these should be disregarded. Health education is thus situated in a grey and confusing world of ambiguity and contradiction which multiplies and complicates dilemmas and makes the formulation of ethically responsible policies and methods very difficult. The identification of overt and covert values, interests and interest groups and decisions about how far these should be colluded and cooperated with—or rejected—lies at the heart of the political tensions within which health education has to operate.

Having identified some themes relevant to ethical reflection on the political tensions surrounding health education, we can move on to examine how these work out in practice, taking as examples the work of the Health Education Council in general and one of its campaigns in particular.

CASE STUDY 1: THE HEALTH EDUCATION COUNCIL

The Health Education Council (HEC) was founded in 1968 by the British Government.[26] It operated as a 'quango'—that is to say that, although government funded, it was an autonomous company limited by guarantee which was given charitable status. The Secretaries of State for Health and Education nominated the 26 members of the HEC, but it was not under the direct control of any government department. This meant it had considerable independence. However, government financial support was not substantial. In 1986–87, the total budget of the HEC was £10 million. Although an equivalent or greater sum may be spent on health education at local level by local and health authorities, this must be compared with an estimated £1 million per week spent on advertising alone by tobacco companies in 1975 and 1989 estimates that the alcohol industry spends £6 million per week on advertising.[27–29]

The ethos of British health education in the 1970s was, by and large, narrow, limited, and individualistic.[15] It harmonized well with governmental perceptions and priorities set out in the consultative document, *Prevention and Health: Everybody's Business* (1976) where statements like the following are to be found:

'The role of the health professions and of government is limited to ensuring that the public have access to such knowledge as is available about the importance of personal habit on health and that at the very least no obstacles are placed in the way of those who decide to act on that knowledge.'[30]

The same document states: 'Much of the responsibility for ensuring his own good health lies with the individual' and affirms the primacy of personal behaviour and attitudes over environmental factors. This kind of thinking lay at the heart of major HEC campaigns like the 'Look after Yourself' Campaign (1978) and the 'Play it Safe' Campaign (1981) which was designed to reduce childhood accidents.[31]

In 1982 David Player was appointed Director-General of the HEC. Coming from the more politicized and militant Scottish Health Education Group, he became increasingly concerned with health promotion understood as doing what has to be done to improve the health of the population and including health education, fiscal action, legal action, action aimed at achieving environmental change, and political action. Player was not alone in recognizing that attaining voluntary attitudinal and behavioural change on the part of individuals by providing 'sound' information was not an adequate health promotion strategy, but he was more confrontational than most in challenging the British government and a range of interest groups to put this wider view across. His experiences expose some of the difficulties and dilemmas which face those who want to actively promote health and to situate health education within this wider vision rather than simply undertaking limited educational campaigns which collude with individualism and 'victim blaming' and which may in fact blur the sociopolitical origins and implications of much illness and disease.

Poverty, Inequality, and Health

One of the most devastating, academically well-founded, and clear findings of social epidemiology to be made public in the last 20 years was the exposure by a

British governmental working party that the incidence of ill-health and disease was inversely related to class position.[19] Thus people in the lowest social classes have higher mortality rates for all diseases (with the exception of breast and ovarian cancer and skin cancer) than people in the highest social classes:

'There are marked inequalities in health between the social classes in Britain ... Mortality tends to rise inversely with falling occupational rank or status, for both sexes and at all ages. At birth and in the first month of life twice as many babies of unskilled manual parents as of professional parents die, and in the next eleven months of life nearly three times as many boys and more than three times as many girls, respectively, die. In the later years of childhood the ratio of deaths in the poorest class falls to between one and a half and two times that of the wealthiest class, but increases again in early adulthood before falling again in middle and old age.'[19]

The authors of *The Black Report* suggested changes in the health and social services costing about two billion pounds to deal with deficiencies in health care provision. They were also quite clear that the battle against inequalities in health has to be situated within a wide strategy to obtain wider social equality and justice. Not surprisingly, this overtly political formulation of a way of combating the inequitable distribution of illness did not find favour with the government of the day, which issued the report in a limited edition on a public holiday weekend in 1980.

As Director-General of the HEC, Player commissioned a follow-up to the original report which confirmed both its diagnosis and solutions when it was published as *The Health Divide* by the HEC in 1987.[32] The introduction to a combined edition of both works tells a fascinating tale of political intrigue with relation to this publication.[19]

It had been planned to launch *The Health Divide* at a press conference in the HEC's offices. At the very last minute, the Chair of the HEC, Sir Brian Bailey, decided to cancel the conference. While not admitting to having been pressurized in any way by government, it is known that a senior civil servant had contacted Sir Brian the night before the launch and circumstantial evidence suggests that he was invited to think again about the wisdom of releasing the report in what looked like being an election year. The upshot was that the report was launched and an 'unofficial' press conference occurred at the offices of the Disability Alliance attended by members of the panel who had compiled it. The Director-General and staff of the HEC who had commissioned the report were forbidden to attend by Sir Brian. All this attracted massive publicity and the report was immediately reprinted because of popular demand.[19]

While this improbable account of attempted government intervention and suppression clearly illustrates the futility and counterproductive nature of heavy-handed action, the primary point of recounting it here is to highlight the controversial nature of health education when it attempts to promote health at all levels of society, to expose the roots of ill-health in the social and political order, and not merely to instruct individuals. Had the HEC not been on the point of dissolution anyway, it is tempting to speculate whether more subtle pressures might not have been brought on it and its senior employees to desist from this kind of politically sensitive exploration and dissemination.

Unemployment and Health

The 1970s and 1980s have seen a rise in research into the effects of unemployment on health. There is now a well-documented literature which makes it clear that unemployment wreaks havoc on the physical and mental health of the population.[33] It is thought that at least 3000 deaths can be directly related to unemployment each year. One study carried out in Edinburgh in 1984 showed that attempted suicide rates in unemployed men, as compared with those in employment, rose very significantly with the amount of time spent out of work. For those unemployed for less than six months attempted suicide rates were 10 times greater than among employed men. This increased to 19 times greater when the time of unemployment was greater than 12 months.[34]

In his previous post as Director of the Scottish Health Education Group (SHEG) in the late 1970s, Player had been aware of research connecting ill-health and unemployment for some years. He was anxious to publicize this trend on the basis of research undertaken by the distinguished American epidemiologist, Harvey Brenner, and so a press conference was called to publicize Brenner's findings. When it became known through the press coverage that Player had become involved in this event, indeed had promoted it, he was called to account by the chair of SHEG at the behest of the Secretary of State for Scotland. It seems likely that he would have been required to resign, but for the fact that he was able to argue that commenting on unemployment and health was simply a matter of his personal medical opinion.

The purpose of this narrative is to emphasize the sensitivity in state-sponsored health education of making any connections at all between social causes of ill-health and their implications for health education and promotion. Government would prefer illness and its causes and together with health education and promotion to be confined to the realm of individual responsibility and behaviour. Those who challenge this view may only be saved by their high professional status.

Anti-Health Forces and their Political Control

Brief mention has already been made of the amounts of money spent by the alcohol and tobacco industries in promoting their products. These interest groups are very powerful in British society. They are designated as anti-health forces or health antagonists for the simple reason that tobacco and alcohol are well known to harm health and cause disease. One hundred thousand premature deaths are caused by the consumption of tobacco products in the United Kingdom each year, yet the industry has consistently refused to admit responsibility for this.[35] Its only defence, if it is one, is to argue that this is a medical matter and as manufacturers, they are not medically competent!

The harm caused by alcohol is greater in social terms than that caused by tobacco, although 20 000 deaths caused by alcohol consumption in one form or another cannot be seen as negligible.[28,29] There is good evidence that the abuse of alcohol is responsible for a majority of crimes relating to violence such as wife battering, baby battering, and homicide. A large number of road and home accidents can also be attributed to alcohol, yet in the last 30 years more alcohol has been sold and consumed in the United Kingdom while its relative cost in real terms is declining.[28,29]

Both the alcohol and tobacco industries indulge in extensive advertising and sponsorship of sporting and cultural events.[36] Although the former has agreed voluntarily that it will not target children or young people, there are 16 football clubs which are sponsored by alcohol firms and players' shirts carry alcohol brand names. Thus, although fans are not allowed to take alcohol into football matches, or allowed to enter if under the influence of drink, they stand watching players advertising alcohol for 90 minutes at a time. Some of these fans are obviously under the legal age where they could purchase alcohol, some are still children. Sportswear firms now produce replica football kit for children as young as 5 years of age. This means that there are young children running around the streets actively promoting alcohol.

Tobacco companies similarly avoid the spirit of voluntary agreements by persuading governments of all political types that advertisements are only concerned with trying to advertise particular brands of cigarette. Advertisements are now increasingly subtle—often they can only be identified as such by a government health warning at the bottom—and they seem to be aiming for subliminal effect on the population. They are increasingly targeted upon the young and women, among whom smoking is on the increase.

Perhaps the chief health antagonist in Britain is not the tobacco or alcohol companies themselves, but the government. The government receives billions of pounds each year from tobacco and alcohol taxes—alcohol contributed 4 billion pounds to the treasury in 1986.[37] Many Members of Parliament (at least 40 declared) have financial interests and consultancies in the tobacco and related industries. Small wonder, then, that a junior health minister who had formerly headed up an alcohol lobby, the Licensed Victuallers' Association, in the House of Commons told David Player early in his Directorship at the HEC that that body could not contribute any money toward Action on Alcohol Abuse, an alliance of medical colleges and others which was partly initiated by HEC concern. More recently (1989) the government has refused to increase duty on alcohol and tobacco in line with the Retail Price Index, thus implicitly encouraging consumption of these products. Indeed, the real price of alcohol in the United Kingdom has been halved in the last 40 years, while consumption has doubled.

How, then, is health education to function effectively when it is sponsored by a body which itself appears to be against the health interests of the greater public whose welfare it was ostensibly elected to protect and which contradicts by its fiscal and other policies what it officially promotes in health education campaigns? In this kind of environment there is a real danger that health education will be perceived as a narrow, cheap, and ineffective tokenism which pre-empts public criticism and outcry about political indifference to promoting health while only being able to do minor things which have limited parameters and results.

Sponsorship

'Health' is a very good word to have associated with any commercial product in contemporary British society. This brings with it political tensions and dilemmas for health educationalists. Not all products are unambiguously good for people. The promotion of health by company sponsorship may cast aspersions and doubts on the truth of the messages being put across as well as determining the content and presentation of messages in certain ways.[38] Indeed, the independence and credibility of a health promotion organization such as HEC may be compromised by the wrong kind of commercial sponsorship. Finally, it must be noted that some of the most affluent and keen sponsors of health promotion and activity are those who sell the most unhealthy products. They wish to clean up their image by positive associations and apparent concern and altruism.

At the same time, however, it must be recognized that not all products are necessarily harmful and that money for health education and promotion is in very short supply from central governmental sources. For this reason, Player proposed the following code for products with which HEC was willing to be positively associated:

1. The organization can pursue associations with commercial bodies when they support its own aims and objectives.
2. The organization will not accept any money or assistance from the tobacco industry or trusts set up with money from the tobacco industry.
3. The organization can work with alcohol companies if the aim is to promote responsible attitudes to drinking alcohol or to encourage wider use and availability of low or non-alcohol drinks.
4. The organization should not have any association with specific branded drugs or dietary supplements or infant feeding formulae.
5. The organization should only collaborate with a pharmaceutical company where the association between a product and the resource being funded is not so close as to be ndistinguishable in the minds of professionals and the public.
6. The organization should only encourage association with food products when the following aims and objectives are promoted:
   (a) a reduction in total fat intake in the diet, especially saturated fats;
   (b) an increase in the consumption of fibre;

(c) a reduction in sugar consumption;

(d) the changes above can be achieved within a diet which meets energy, mineral, and vitamin requirements, is widely obtainable and reasonably priced;

(e) the avoidance of special vitamins and other dietary supplements;

(f) reduction of salt intake.

7. No commercial association should impair the good name and standing of the organisation.

Despite giving considerable care and attention to these guidelines, the HEC has been criticized for accepting commercial sponsorship. Writing of sponsorship by Allied Bakeries of the 1985 'Great British Fun Run', Naidoo notes

'This sponsorship gave valuable funding for the event, but also, inevitably, affected the content of the campaign. Thus the educational message to "eat more fibre" became translated into the selling message "eat more Allinson's wholemeal and Hi-bran bread". Sponsorship affects not only content, but also credibility...It is likely that sponsorship gives professional legitimacy to a product, so that people will think more highly of Allied Bakeries because their product is associated with the HEC. But it is equally likely that some of the HEC's credibility as an impartial adviser on health could be jeopardised by such an association with a commercial company.'[31]

There is no easy way of balancing losses and gains in relation to commercial sponsorship and funding of this kind. It is yet another aspect of the socioeconomic and political tensions which surround health educators as they seek the welfare of the British people.

On 21 November 1986, it was unexpectedly announced that the Health Education Council was to be disbanded to be replaced in April 1987 with a new Health Education Authority (HEA). The new Authority was to be a Special Health Authority, directly responsible to the Secretary of State for Health like all other English health authorities and with members appointed directly by him. The independence of the HEC was not to be retained and, in future, the Department of Health was to be consulted as to the detail and subject matter of all campaigns for its approval. The main stated reason for the change was that a new, larger, and more vigorous organization was needed to head up the dissemination of health information in the light of the AIDS epidemic which was just beginning to become visible as a threat to public health at that time. Unofficially, many wondered if the occasion was being used to get rid of a body which had become too keen on making social and political connnections between disease, ill-health, and health promotion.[39]

If the sincerest form of flattery from an opponent is that they try to eliminate or silence you, the members and staff of the HEC may feel that they did have some political impact and that not all their health promotion responses were simply individualistic or analgesic. And if the HEC had to fight for the promotion of the people's health with one arm tied behind its back because it had to compromise with government and other powerful interest groups, it is quite clear that the HEA has both arms tied behind its back. Recent anxieties (1988) about salmonella and the purity of the food chain, engendered chiefly by a junior government minister who has subsequently lost her job at the Department of Health, have not elicited any guidance to the public from the HEA, despite widespread public alarm. A casual enquiry to the Authority from one of the authors in April 1989 was met with a slightly embarrassed response: 'Yes, we are concerned about it, but we are very busy with AIDS and it is a very controversial area.' So controversial, in fact, that the British government has done all in its power to soothe chicken farmers with compensation of £3 million and to stifle public knowledge and debate.

CASE STUDY 2: THE POLITICS OF HEALTH INFORMATION

The political tensions and ethical dilemmas confronting health education are also revealed at a different level in a study of the politics of health information undertaken by Farrant and Russell in relation to one particular HEC campaign, 'Beating Heart Disease' in 1984.[4] Farrant and Russell assert that the content and style of communication together with the style and manner of production of the booklet, *Beating Heart Disease* epitomizes the conventional, individual behaviour-oriented approach to health education. This approach is characterized as (i) 'victim-blaming' in orientation, failing to take account of social determinants of ill-health; (ii) 'top-down' in planning, so that the health concerns, experiences, and self-defined information needs of target audience are ignored in favour of professional preoccupations and concerns; (iii) prescriptive in style, so that the 'active-and-dominant expert, passive-and-dependent client' model is reinforced and people are not encouraged to act individually and collectively to take control of their own health.

Farrant and Russell start their analysis by pointing out that the causes of coronary heart disease (CHD) are many. Scientific research itself tends to suggest that relations between people and between people and their social environment are at least as important as individual high-risk behaviours such as poor eating or smoking. Social, environmental, and stress factors need to be changed if good health is to be encouraged, but this was ignored in the information provided in *Beating Heart Disease*.

Beating Heart Disease had to be produced in a very short time to fit in with complementary media programmes being broadcast by the BBC. This meant that the booklet was put together by a very small number of people. They were mainly consultant physicians and there was little input by health educationalists. There was no time to research widely to get examples from all parts of society (so most examples in the booklet related to white middle-class people) and the booklet could not be pretested or piloted with the public before release. Data on the depth and complexity of lay knowledge, beliefs, and values on CHD aetiology and prevention were thus ignored.

Farrant and Russell point out that important and controversial political (in the widest sense of the term) assumptions underlay the production of *Beating Heart Disease*:

1. The assumption that it is not the role of HEC publications to challenge government dictated social policy (so references to social and environmental change were excluded in the final version of the booklet).
2. The assumption that HEC publications should reflect a consensus of mainstream medical opinion (so multiple explanations were excluded).
3. Assumptions were made about the information needs of the target audience (so it was assumed that the publication should be short and simple, aimed at those who had a reading ability no higher than that of a tabloid newspaper without any substantive research into whether this was appropriate, and professional assumptions about the intellectual abilities of people in lower social classes were acted upon).
4. The assumption that the HEC must 'sell health' by analogy with marketing a product or commodity to consumers (so adopting advertising methods which try to put across one simple point in a prescriptive style and thus falling into a 'propagandist' and pragmatic mode of communication).

Outlining lay perspectives on CHD, its aetiology, and prevention, Farrant and Russell highlight the finding that lay people had a very complex view and believed that there were many relevant factors. Lay people could, for example, see that stress was an important factor, as were environmental conditions. To them, being asked to believe one simple message was incredible—the credibility of 'expert' knowledge was undermined by its oversimplification. In the same way, lay people could see that it was not solely their responsibility to change and were all too aware of the difficulties of doing this, given their conflicting responsibilities. For example, women are not necessarily free to feed their families differently if 'healthy' food is too expensive or if their families will not eat it.[23] Likewise, smoking might be an important aspect of preserving family mental health which can be conceived as a higher ethical value than simply preventing individual CHD.

Farrant and Russell conclude that the view of CHD put forward in the *Beating Heart Disease* leaflet 'ignores or minimizes the role of the social environment in which individuals live, and thereby, ultimately reduces health education's own chances of effectiveness'. They argue for a broader and social perspective which is more effective and more intellectually honest:

'In supporting a social perspective, we are not denying the importance of individuals in CHD prevention, or as recipients of health information, but rather are calling for a style of health education that is more intellectually honest in its reflection of epidemiological evidence, and more sensitive, appropriate and empowering to the lives of the individuals it addresses.'

Whether or not one agrees with all aspects of Farrant and Russell's analysis of one particular HEC booklet, it cannot be denied that it highlights in a very helpful way many of the specific practical political tensions facing state-sponsored health education today.

CONCLUSION

Like politics itself, health education is the art of the possible. Grossly underfunded and resourced, health educators as individuals and as a group have a central and crucially important job in contemporary society. They are regarded as significant enough for governments to lay down strict guidelines for their activity and for powerful interest groups to seek their approbation and association. As with any significant and important function, health education is fraught with ambiguities and tensions. Doubtless, many health educators would be only too happy to be less dependent on professional medical knowledge, to be more contextual and flexible in the messages they enunciate, to have more regard to lay perceptions of illness, to use methods which enhance and reinforce people's ability to take control of their own lives and define their own good health. To the extent that health education is narrowly professionalized, ineffectual, propagandist, 'victim-blaming', or simply as an apology for the vital complementary task of tackling social and environmental issues, health educators often feel ashamed and regretful themselves. Who, after all, is in a better position to see all the factors which bear on ill-health and disease prevention than this group of people?

Marxist critics will not be surprised at the tensions explored in this chapter. To them, health education is merely one more part of the control apparatus of the state. It is therefore bound to be essentially oppressive and ideological as it seeks to promote the interests of capital and powerful groups in society over those of the poor—those who disproportionately experience environmentally and socially caused ill-health and have least chance of changing their circumstances for the better.[40-42] While recognizing some truth in this analysis, it cannot be accepted in full. Even Marxists acknowledge that the capitalist social order is riven with contradictions, some of which favour the real interests of the majority of the people. Health education can be something more than an opiate for the masses. It can authoritatively and effectively challenge health antagonists and conspiracies against the social and environmental causes of illness being recognized, as the demise of the HEC witnesses all too clearly.

It must, however, be recognized that good, comprehensive, and responsible health education—like many other ethically respectable activities—requires finance, human resources, time, and relative independence from state or commercial interference. Health education will retain an aura of hasty expediency and pragmatism until these conditions are more adequately met. Whether these conditions will be met is, of course, a political decision.

Health educators and authorities maintained by the state are constantly involved in important dilemmas and issues of the kind outlined above. It is always possible to take a 'purist' line and decide that health education is compromised in such a way that it cannot possibly help people; indeed, that it disguises and distorts the nature of reality. People who believe this presumably cease to be state-employed health educators. Those who stay, however, have to wrestle with the ambiguities of their role, work, and messages amid a complex and confusing social and political reality. Many compromises present themselves and there appear to be many slippery ethical and political slopes to be negotiated. For those with the right sense of balance and commitment perhaps it is possible not to slide right down to the bottom of the slopes precipitately but, like the expert skier, to use and negotiate them so the true health education needs of the public are in fact served, at least some of the time.

REFERENCES

1. Seedhouse, D. *Health: The Foundations for Achievement*. Chichester: Wiley, 1986.
2. Wilson, M. *Health is for People*. London: Darton, Longman and Todd, 1974.
3. Cribb, A. Politics and health in the school curriculum. In: *The Politics of Health Education*. Rodmell, S. and Watt, A. (eds.). London: Routledge and Kegan Paul, 1986.
4. Farrant, W. and Russell, J. *The Politics of Health Information*. London: Institute of Education, University of London, 1986.
5. O'Neill, O. *Faces of Hunger*. London: Allen and Unwin, 1986.
6. Lukes, S. *Individualism*. Oxford: Blackwell, 1973.
7. Watt, A. Community health education. In: *The Politics of Health Education*, Rodmell, S. and Watt, A. (eds.). London: Routledge and Kegan Paul, 1986.
8. Johnson, T. *Professions and Power*. London: Macmillan, 1972.
9. Freidson, E. *Profession of Medicine*. New York: Dodd, Mead, 1975.
10. Waitzking, H. and Waterman, B. *The Exploitation of Illness in Capitalist Society*. Indianapolis: Bobbs-Merrill, 1974.
11. Cornwell, J. *Hard-earned Lives*. London: Tavistock, 1984.
12. Currer, C. and Stacey, M. (eds.). *Concepts of Health, Illness and Disease*. Leamington Spa: Berg, 1986.
13. Helman, C. *Culture, Health and Illness*. Bristol: Wright, 1984.
14. Wilding, P. *Professional Power and Social Welfare*. London: Routledge and Kegan Paul, 1982.
15. Rodmell, S. and Watt, A. Conventional health education: problems and possibilities. In: *The Politics of Health Education*. Rodmell, S. and Watt, A. (eds.). London: Routledge and Kegan Paul, 1986.
16. Campbell, A. *Medicine, Health and Justice*. Edinburgh: Churchill Livingstone, 1978.
17. Miller, D. *Social Justice*. Oxford: Oxford University Press, 1976.
18. Plant, R., Lesser, H. and Taylor-Gooby, P. *Political Philosophy and Social Welfare*. London: Routledge and Kegan Paul, 1980.
19. Black, D., Morris, J., Smith, C. *et al*. *Inequalities in Health*. London: Penguin, 1988.
20. Tawney, R. *Equality*. London: Unwin, 1964.
21. Le Grand, J. *The Strategy of Inequality*. London: George Allen and Unwin, 1982.
22. Raphael, D. *Problems of Political Philosophy*. London: Macmillan, 1976.
23. Charles, N. and Kerr, M. Issues of responsibility and control in the feeding of families.

In: *The Politics of Health Education*. Rodmell, S. and Watt, A. (eds.). London: Routledge and Kegan Paul, 1986.
24. Pattison, S. *Alive and Kicking: Towards a Practical Theology of Illness and Healing*. London: SCM Press, 1989.
25. Plamenatz, J. *Ideology*. London: Macmillan, 1971.
26. Levitt, R. and Wall, J. *The Reorganised National Health Service*. London: Croom Helm, 1984.
27. Doyal, L. *The Political Economy of Health*. London: Pluto, 1979.
28. Royal College of Psychiatrists. *Alcohol: Our Favourite Drug*. London: Tavistock, 1986.
29. Royal College of Physicians. *A Great and Growing Evil*. London: Tavistock, 1987.
30. Department of Health and Social Security. *Prevention and Health*. London: Her Majesty's Stationery Office, 1976.
31. Naidoo, J. Limits to individualism. In: *The Politics of Education*. Rodmell, S. and Watt, A. (eds.). London: Routledge and Kegan Paul, 1986.
32. Whitehead, M. *The Health Divide*. London: Health Education Council, 1987.
33. Smith, R. *Unemployment and Health*. Oxford: Oxford University Press, 1987.
34. Platt, S. and Kreitman, N. Unemployment and parasuicide in Edinburgh 1968–1982. *Br Med J* 1986; **289**: 1029–1032.
35. Smith, A. (ed.). *The Nation's Health*. London: King's Fund, 1988.
36. Steele, D. Advertising. *Action on Alcohol Abuse Review* Jan–Feb. 1989: 17–24.
37. Robinson, J. *On the Demon Drink*. London: Mitchell Beazley, 1988.
38. Editorial. Taking money from the devil. *Br Med J* 1982; **282**: 271.
39. Alleway, L. Is Fowler taming the HEC? *Hlth Service J* 1986; **96**: 1268–1269.
40. Miliband, R. *The State in Capitalist Society*. London: Quartet, 1973.
41. Navarro, V. *Medicine under Capitalism*. New York: Prodist, 1976.
42. Navarro, V. *Class Struggle, the State and Medicine*. London: Martin Robertson, 1978.

CHAPTER 6

The Role of Organized Medicine in the Ethics of Health Education and Health Promotion

OLE K. HARLEM

'A wise man ought to realize that health is his most valuable possession and learn how to treat his illnesses by his own judgment.'

(Hippocrates[1])

SUMMARY

The main objective of this chapter is to shed light on the role of organized medicine in the ethics of health education and health promotion. The role of organized medicine is a difficult and dual one for it has to protect not only the interests of the doctors but those of the patients as well. Despite this conflict, however, organized medicine has achieved much in the field of medical ethics up to now, especially as far as health education is concerned.

INTRODUCTION

The objective of this chapter is to describe and explain the role of organized medicine in the ethics of health education. This will be shown by the examples referred to which will also illustrate the important role organized medicine must play in the years to come, when health education, health promotion, and not least the development of modern biotechnology will make increasing demands on medical ethics. Some relevant statements and resolutions from the World Medical Association (WMA) are presented as appendices to the chapter. The role of organized medicine is also very important as far as the implementation of basic ethical rules is concerned because such rules must be accepted not only by

Ethics in Health Education
Edited by S. Doxiadis. ©1990 John Wiley & Sons Ltd

physicians but by society as well. The achievement of all these goals will not be easy for society has undergone great changes over recent years and the amount of new knowledge has increased significantly. This change is reflected, inter alia, by the presence today of over 40 medical specialties in my country, Norway, and by the fact that there exist almost 100 different categories of health personnel. These facts make it quite clear that the various bodies which represent organized medicine will very often have to be unconventional and be prepared to depart from tradition and to follow new paths.

INFLUENCE OF THE DOCTOR ON MEDICAL ETHICS

Let us first take a look at the role of the doctor. Traditionally doctors have been occupied primarily with diagnosis and treatment of illnesses and they have often been accused of being more interested in diseases than in sick people. This is a plausible complaint since disease has been the dominant concept in medicine for many centuries. As disease has been more or less defined as the 'deviation from a certain norm', it is not surprising that doctors, influenced by this generalized approach, tend to focus more on the disease than on the individual patient. However, I believe this to be an oversimplification. In my own student days I recall that many of our best teachers (serving as our models) were greatly involved with sick people and not only with diseases. This is also true of most of the colleagues I have met and worked with during a long professional life. It is, however, a fact that biotechnological development, increased specialization, and the splitting up of responsibility have led to poorer contact between doctors and patients and lack of emphasis on bedside manner—developments which the mass media have not been slow to exploit.

How do I envisage the role of the doctor in the future? We will certainly need doctors with knowledge and skills in diagnosis and treatment of disease. But as a profession we must realize that the *prevention* of disease and the *preservation* of health take on an ever-increasing importance. Prevention and preservation are closely related to health education and a very important thing to remember about health education is that doctors should take account of the individual not only as an entity but also in interaction with his environment in the broadest sense. Since it is generally accepted that lifestyle diseases have a decisive influence on human health, we obviously need doctors who work in preventive medicine in all its aspects. Because of their solid basic training doctors can become good health educators provided they acquire the necessary supplementary competence. But another important point must be also borne in mind: the public today are much better educated than before and people have the right to be properly informed about illness and health and about the various factors which affect their lives. Only if the information given to them is full and unbiased can they play an active part in the decision processes concerning their own health. For this reason, health educators with a medical training (undergraduate, graduate, and postgraduate) adapted to the needs of our present society and its requirements should not only be ready to shift from a curative to a preventive role but should also be ready to respect the basic principles of medical ethics—autonomy, beneficence, and justice.

THE NEW DIMENSIONS OF MEDICAL ETHICS

This change in the role or roles of doctors does not affect only professional knowledge and skills but professional behaviour as well. Medical ethics acquire today a new dimension. In my days as a medical student and young practitioner medical ethics was a notion with very little content. We had heard about Hippocrates and the Hippocratic Oath, but I had not realized the importance of these matters until I came into contact with organized medicine and was elected Member of Council of The World Medical Association. One of the first acts of The World Medical Association, when formed in 1947, was to produce a modern restatement of the Hippocratic Oath, known as the Declaration of Geneva (see Appendix C).

Far earlier, in 1849, a Committee on Medical Ethics had been formed in Great Britain; this was a forerunner to the present Central Ethical Committee, which is empowered under the articles and byelaws of the British Medical Association.

In Norway ethical rules are an integral part of the articles and byelaws of the Norwegian Medical Association. These ethical rules have focused primarily on the relationship between patients and doctors, on the doctors' professional behaviour, and on the need for loyalty to colleagues.

In an article in the *New England Journal of Medicine* on the definition and teaching of medical ethics, Chapman uses as his starting point the Ethical Codex of the American Medical Association.[2] He asks for changes in the principles of medical codices in medical societies. He wants them to be less doctor- and more patient-oriented. The paternalism which dominates most of the ethical rules laid down by medical associations should be replaced by rules which ascertain patients' rights to information and co-determination. We should move away from ethical rules that are more or less dominated by etiquette for doctors. In the light of Chapman's observations I looked at the ethical rules of the Norwegian Medical Association. It must be admitted that they are still very much doctor-oriented: a doctor shall, a doctor shall not... Very little is said directly about the patient's rights although they are implicit in some of the paragraphs.

The British Medical Association has been very active in the field of medical ethics in the last decades. In 1988 their *Handbook of Medical Ethics*, which was first printed in 1984, was thoroughly revised and published under the title *Philosophy and Practice of Medical Ethics*.[3] The book, and in particular the chapter called 'Continuing ethical dilemmas—no consensus view', gives an excellent overview of various medical ethical problems. Very useful also is a chapter on ethical codes and statements, beginning with the Hippocratic Oath and ending with the European Union of General Practitioners' (URMO) statement on Medical Confidentiality in Relation to the Use of Modern Methods of Communication (EDP) in Medicine presented in Amsterdam in May 1979. It is a little disappointing, however, that the doctor's role in health education and health promotion and the medical ethical implications of this are barely touched upon in the book. If medical associations are to play a key role in this area, a move from doctor dominated to patient- and society-oriented ethical rules, as proposed by Chapman, is essential.

These efforts show clearly that organized medicine has realized the importance of ethics in medicine and health education and promotion. Today many traditional values in medicine are being questioned, and a more serious concentration on the ethics of health matters, including health education might help people restore their lost faith in the medical world. All medical organizations are working hard in this direction.

THE WORLD MEDICAL ASSOCIATION

The World Medical Association (WMA) was founded in Paris on 18 September 1947. Its headquarters are located in Ferney-Voltaire, France, and Dr Andre Wynen serves as Secretary-General. Forty-six national medical associations are members of the WMA. In order to qualify for membership, national medical associations must be non-governmental associations of physicians, representative of physicians in their own countries. These member-associations are joined together to work for the achievement of the highest international standards in medical education medical sciences, medical art, medical ethics, and health care for people all over the world. The WMA is organized into six regions: Africa, Asia, Europe, North America, Pacific, and Latin America. Assembly meetings are held annually to act on the business of the WMA and between these assembly meetings, WMA activities are directed by the WMA Council. Various committees on medical ethics, socio-medical affairs, finance, and planning are also assisting the Council.

Worldwide, the WMA has been the voice of physicians in the shaping of international codes of medical ethics. Medical ethics will continue to command its attention as progress generates new issues and creates the need to modify existing declarations and codes. These declarations and codes have been widely promulgated and serve as guidelines for national medical associations and governmental legislation throughout the world. The British Medical Association in its *Handbook of Medical Ethics*,[3] emphasizes the role of the WMA and rightly so, because, apart from the Declaration of Geneva in 1947, several other declarations and statements have been issued since then.

The Declaration of Geneva (revised at Sydney in 1968 and Venice in 1983) is a modern version of the Hippocratic Oath. This Declaration was followed by another, known as the WMA's International Code of Medical Ethics, adopted in London in 1949 (see Appendix D). Another very important Declaration is the Code of Ethics on human experimentation, drawn up in 1964 and amended by the 29th World Medical Assembly in Helsinki in 1975 and by the World Medical Assembly in Venice in 1983. This declaration has had great impact on human experimentation and has served as a starting point for establishing ethical committees in various countries to scrutinize research projects on human beings. On the whole, practice has shown that the statements and resolutions adopted by WMA have had an impact far beyond the WMA membership. The Helsinki Declaration, for example, has been adopted not only by the WMA countries, but is also recommended by the World Health Organization and thereby accepted by most countries in the world. Some years ago the Nordic countries, the Netherlands, and later Great Britain left the WMA for political reasons. They continued, however, to cooperate with the WMA in ethical matters, especially in the revision of the Helsinki Declaration.

The activity of the WMA in the area of medical ethics does not end there. Very recently I received a letter from the WMA which included one declaration concerning the Access to Health Care and three other statements adopted by the World Medical Assembly in September 1988.

The first statement refers to Health Hazards of Tobacco Products (see Appendix A). The implications of this rather strong statement affect not only health areas but social, commercial, and financial fields as well. Nonetheless, it is essential that the medical profession make it clear where it stands in such an important matter. In many countries statistics show that smoking habits among doctors are changing for the better. In Norway less than 20% of doctors are smokers today. It would not be unreasonable to believe that credit for this development should be given to the Norwegian National Medical Association for the strong position it has taken against smoking. Important as this is, consequences for society are even more significant. We all know the power of example!

The second statement refers to the role of the physician in environmental and demographic issues (see Appendix B). At last, we seem to realize that we cannot continue to contaminate our globe in the way we have done for generations now, if we want to survive. In my opinion this declaration touches the core of the question. Much of what we have done hitherto, and are still doing, in health education and health promotion merely scratches the surface of these problem areas. The strong and clear standpoint which the WMA has taken in this controversial area is a token of foresight and courage. It is our responsibility now to take up the gauntlet thrown by the WMA. Although there will be differences of opinion as to how these problems should be solved, it is time to move from talk and discussion to action. In this process medical associations and national and international scientific societies have an important role to play, trying to use their influence to persuade politicians and other decision-makers to act before it is too late.

The third statement concerns AIDS—one of the touchest challenges in the modern history of mankind. In the mass media and among professionals, discussion on AIDS continues, quite often characterized more by emotion than by common sense. We cannot expect to arrive at a consensus of opinion on the ethical aspects of AIDS. Nevertheless, it is important that the medical profession tries to take a stand in such an important matter. The WMA has issued two statements on AIDS. The first was adopted in October 1987 and it states in part: 'Patients with AIDS and those who test positively for the antibody to the AIDS virus must be provided with appropriate medical care and should not be treated unfairly or suffer from arbitrary or irrational discrimination in their daily lives. Physicians have a long and honoured tradition of tending to patients afflicted with contagious diseases with compassion and courage. This tradition must be continued throughout the AIDS epidemic.' The second statement, on the professional responsibilities of those treating AIDS patients, was adopted at the 40th World Assembly in Vienna, Austria, in September 1988.

THE RELATIONSHIP OF THE WMA WITH OTHER ORGANIZATIONS

So far, I have stressed the role of the WMA in the area of medical ethics and health promotion and I have also presented some of the more than 25 codes, resolutions, and statements on medical ethics adopted by the WMA since 1947. Three important questions may now arise:

1. What are WMA's relations with governmental agencies?
2. What are WMA's relations with the World Health Organization?
3. Are all these resolutions, codes and statements getting the attention they deserve?

I will try to answer these questions one by one.

(1) WMA's relations with governmental agencies nationally and internationally are good, in particular with organizations such as the United Nations Educational, Scientific and Cultural Organization (UNESCO), the Union of Industries of the European Community (UNICEF), the International Labour Organization (ILO), and the International Social Security Association (ISSA). There is a continuing exchange of communications and literature and consultation on projects between these organizations and the WMA. The World Medical Organization sends observers to their meetings and they are represented at WMA meetings. Lately, UNICEF has been keeping regular contact with WMA because of the latter's Infant Health Project now being implemented in Indonesia and Thailand.

(2) Some years ago the WMA lost its non-governmental status with the World Health Organization. However, since Dr Hiroshi Nakajima took over as Director-General of the World Health Organization, relations have improved remarkably. On 7 April 1989, in his message for World Health Day, Dr Nakajima said: 'I have decided to devote World Health Day 1989 to the theme of communication for health and I should like to make a solemn appeal to all those responsible for informing, for educating or for creating social dialogue—the cause of health needs you...'.

(3) World Medical Association declarations, statements, and resolutions are making the impact they deserve and are highly respected, quoted, and followed by individuals and national and international organizations alike. The incredibly rapid medical advances and progress and the related medical ethics problems

they pose to the medical profession have motivated people, institutions, and governments to resort to guidelines which are available thanks to WMA. The World Medical Association has acted on topics such as biomedical research in man, family planning, death, therapeutic abortion, computers in medicine, torture and maltreatment of detainees, psychotropic drugs, pollution, capital punishment, rights of the patient, terminal illness, boxing, tobacco health hazards, physicians' role in environmental and demographic issues, access to health care, child abuse and neglect, sports medicine, live organ trade, *in vitro* fertilization, euthanasia, human organ transplantation, AIDS, genetic counselling and genetic engineering, and fetal tissue transplantation. Ethical problems relevant to health education and health promotion will certainly be dealt with more specifically in the near future.

The best and most direct channel for the WMA to influence governments and politicians to react to its declarations is the national member associations, and here it must be stressed that not only have the more affluent and powerful medical associations been an important and vital instrument. Small member associations such as those in Chile, Philippines, Fiji, Malta, Portugal, Panama and Colombia have also done a remarkable job in making WMA documents known to their respective governments. In short, WMA declarations and in particular the International Code of Medical Ethics, the Declaration of Helsinki, and the Declaration of Tokyo have had a huge global effect on governments, the United Nations, the World Health Organization, the Council of Europe, and on most of the largest and most prestigious pharmaceutical firms, and, most importantly, have served as a basis for subsequent documents adopted by the World Health Organization, the United Nations, the Council of Europe, and so on.

CONCLUSIONS

The role of international organizations (medical or non-medical) has been often questioned. They have been accused of being too slow and too costly. They have been accused of serving personal ambitions and of becoming political battlegrounds. They have been accused of simply representing and reinforcing the status of the powerful people and countries. Although these complaints do not lack some truth, it would be unfair not to focus on the more positive aspects of such national and international medical bodies. Their function may present certain problems but their utility is unquestionable. As most modern societies are organized by laws and regulations it is not at all surprising that medicine is following the same path. Organized medicine is a completely natural development and product of the kind of society we live in; people realize that only by being united at national or international level can they achieve their goals, one of the most important of which is health. In this chapter I have argued that organized medicine should play a key role in the formulation of medical ethics in health promotion. This role presents a special difficulty: health promotion is usually directed towards a whole population in a certain society or country whereas medical ethics most often refers to the individual patient. The existing declarations are sets of laws and regulations which would be completely meaningless if they were not accompanied by some moral rules as well, such as the autonomy of the individual patient, the duty to tell the truth, and many others. The existing medical codes, therefore, will be meaningless if every doctor does not take into consideration not only the relevant legal principles but the moral ones as well. As Kennedy has stated '...the principles by reference to which we organize our lives and decide what we ought or ought not to do, are not the preserve of any one group'.[4] It is not always sufficient to abide by some legal rules; it is necessary also to obey another kind of code. As the Declaration of Geneva says: '...I will not use my medical knowledge contrary to the laws of humanity.'

APPENDIX A

World Medical Association Statement on Health Hazards of Tobacco Products

Adopted by the 40th World Medical Assembly at Vienna, Austria, September 1988

There is overwhelming and incontrovertible scientific evidence that the use of tobacco products is related to serious adverse health consequences in those who use such products. Furthermore, irritating and harmful substances from smoking tobacco may impose a health burden on non-smokers who are in proximity to smokers.

Assuming that action has not been taken, WMA urges the National Medical Associations and all physicians to take the following actions to help reduce the health hazards related to smoking and other use of tobacco products:

1. Adopt a policy position opposing smoking and the use of tobacco products, and publicize the policy so adopted.
2. Prohibit smoking and the use of tobacco products at all meetings of the National Medical Association. For many years WMA has had a standing order (No.24) that prohibits smoking in meeting rooms where WMA meetings are being conducted.
3. Develop, support, and participate in programmes to educate the profession and the public to the health hazards of tobacco products. Education programmes directed specifically at children and young adults to avoid the use of tobacco products are particularly important. Programmes for non-smokers and non-users of smokeless tobacco products aimed at avoidance are as necessary as education aimed at convincing smokers to cease the use of tobacco products.
4. Encourage individual physicians to be role models (by not using tobacco products) and spokesmen for the campaign to educate the public about the deleterious effects on health resulting from the use of tobacco products. Ask all hospitals and health facilities to prohibit smoking on their premises.
5. Advocate the enactment and enforcement of laws that:
    (a) require warnings about health hazards to be printed on all packages in which tobacco products are sold and in all advertising and promotional materials for tobacco products.
    (b) limit smoking in public buildings, commercial airliners, schools, hospitals, clinics, and other health facilities.

(c) impose limitations on advertising and sales promotion of tobacco products.
(d) regulate or prohibit the importation of tobacco products.
(e) prohibit the sales of cigarettes and other tobacco products to children and adolescents.
(f) prohibit smoking on all commercial airline flights within national borders and on all international commercial airline flights, and prohibit the sale of tax-free tobacco products at airports.
(g) prohibit all governments' subsidies for tobacco and tobacco products.
(h) provide for research into the prevalence of use of tobacco products and the effects of tobacco products on the health status of the population, and develop educational programmes for the public about the health hazards of tobacco use.
(i) prohibit the promotion, distribution, and sale of any new forms of tobacco products that are not currently available.
(j) increase taxation of tobacco products, using the increase revenues for health care measures.

APPENDIX B

World Medical Association Declaration on The Role of Physicians in Environmental and Demographic Issues

Adopted by the 40th World Medical Assembly, Vienna, Austria, September 1988

Introduction

The effective practice of medicine requires that physicians and their professional associations address environmental and demographic issues that can influence the health status of both individuals and large populations. Broadly speaking these issues all concern the quality and availability of those resources that are necessary for the maintenance of health and ultimately for life itself. Specifically, environmental issues have four dimensions that in the long and short term influence health:

A. The need to halt the degradation of the environment so that resources necessary for life and health, e.g. clean air and water, can be available to all. The persistent chemical and waste contamination of our fresh water supplies and of our atmosphere with hydrocarbons can have severe medical consequences.
B. The need to control the use of non-renewable resources, e.g. top soil and oil, so that they can provide benefits to further generations.
C. The need to utilize reasonable and universal family planning methods so that sustainable society is maintained and medical resources remain available.
D. The need to mobilize resources across national boundaries in order to develop broad, internationally based solutions to these broad, internationally based problems.

The primary objective of this declaration is to increase the awareness for maintaining the necessary balance between environmental resources on the one hand and the biological and social requirements for health on the other. From the perspective of the physician, neither exponential population growth nor the irresponsible destruction of the environment is acceptable. Throughout the world, organized medicine should stand as an advocate for resolving these issues.

Principles

1. As an element in their representation of physicians, medical societies should consider environmental issues. This consideration can include the identification of problems that have a particular local urgency; efforts to improve the enforcement of already existing laws on environmental issues; and the identification of health issues that have their roots in environmental problems.
2. Medical societies should promote family planning measures that are medically and ethically sound. The goal of such measures will not be to inhibit the personal autonomy of individuals but rather to enrich the quality of life for all family members and for the continuation of life on the planet.
3. The WMA should serve as an international forum on the medical impact on environmental and demographic issues and should provide a forum for coordinating the international efforts by physicians and medical societies on the many such issues that must be addressed internationally.

APPENDIX C

Declaration of Geneva

(as amended at Sydney, 1968)

At the time of being admitted as a member of the medical profession:

I will solemnly pledge myself to consecrate my life to the service of humanity;

I will give to my teachers the respect and gratitude which is their due;

I will practise my profession with conscience and dignity;

The health of my patient will be my first consideration;

I will respect the secrets which are confided in me, even after the patient has died;

I will maintain by all the means in my power the honour and the noble traditions of the medical profession;

My colleagues will be my brothers;

I will not permit considerations of religion, nationality, race, party politics or social standing to intervene between my duty and my patient;

I will maintain the utmost respect for human life from the time of conception; even under threat, I will not use my medical knowledge contrary to the laws of humanity.

I make these promises solemnly, freely and upon my honour.

APPENDIX D

International Code of Medical Ethics

Duties of Doctors in General
A DOCTOR MUST always maintain the highest standards of professional conduct.
A DOCTOR MUST practise his profession uninfluenced by motives of profit.
THE FOLLOWING PRACTICES are deemed unethical:

(a) Any self-advertisement except such as is expressly authorized by the national code of medical ethics.
(b) Collaboration in any form of medical service in which the doctor does not have professional independence.

(c) Receiving any money in connection with services rendered to a patient other than a proper professional fee, even with the knowledge of the patient.

ANY ACT OR ADVICE which could weaken physical or mental resistance of a human being may be used only in his interest.
A DOCTOR IS ADVISED to use great caution in divulging discoveries of new techniques of treatment.
A DOCTOR SHOULD certify or testify only to that which he has personally verified.

Duties of Doctors to the Sick
A DOCTOR MUST always bear in mind the obligation of preserving human life.
A DOCTOR OWES to his patient complete loyalty and all the resources of his science. Whenever an examination or treatment is beyond his capacity he should summon another doctor who has the necessary ability.
A DOCTOR SHALL preserve absolute secrecy on all he knows about his patients because of the confidence entrusted in him.
A DOCTOR MUST give emergency care as a humanitarian duty unless he is assured that others are willing and able to give such care.

Duties of Doctors to Each Other
A DOCTOR OUGHT to behave to his colleagues as he would have them behave to him.
A DOCTOR MUST NOT entice patients from his colleagues.
A DOCTOR MUST OBSERVE the principles of the 'The Declaration of Geneva' approved by the World Medical Association.

REFERENCES

1. Chadwick, J. and Mann, W.N. *The Medical Works of Hippocrates*. Oxford: Blackwell, 1950.
2. Chapman, C.P. On the definition and teaching of medical ethics. *N Engl J Med* 1979; **301**: 630–634.
3. *Philosophy and Practice of Medical Ethics*. London: British Medical Association, 1988.
4. Kennedy, I. Unmasking medicine. The Reith Lectures. *The Listener*, 27 November, 1980.

Note: All codes, declaration, statements, and resolutions on medical ethics adopted by the WMA, can be obtained by writing to The World Medical Association, 28 Avenue des Alpes, 01210 Ferney-Voltaire, France.

CHAPTER 7

The Journalist as Health Educator

JEAN-DANIEL FLAYSAKIER

SUMMARY

Health topics are attracting ever-increasing attention from the media. And this appetite for medical stories has brought newspapers, radio stations, and television networks into fierce competition to be the first to deliver the story. This competition is not always handled professionally from the scientific point of view—many so-called medical journalists lack a medical or biological background and this lack of knowledge together with the time constraints always present in the media world can be ethically dangerous. Medical journalism, however, is a part of public health education today. Whether we like it or not, the public tends to believe what they read or hear or see in a reputable media source. Given the new challenges in health—such as, for example, the AIDS epidemic—it is no exaggeration to say that medical journalists are vital players in the field of public health. It thus becomes urgent to define stricter ethical guidelines and standards for the treatment of health topics in the media so that all concerned play by the same rules.

INTRODUCTION

It is clear today that the medical community can no longer afford to ignore the growing importance of the media in the practice of medicine. This importance is nourished by the expectations of a public fascinated by advances in medicine and biology and by other, perhaps less obvious, factors. There is competition between the individual branches of the media themselves which can lead to conclusions arrived at too hastily, and sometimes taken too far. There is pressure from commercial firms who 'choose' a particular journalist to announce a scoop in the pharmaceutical or biological field with its eventual consequences in the financial markets. And there is also a desire on the part of some doctors to achieve recognition through the media. All these factors inevitably influence our knowledge

Ethics in Health Education
Edited by S. Doxiadis. ©1990 John Wiley & Sons Ltd

of medicine. And there are dangers. Journalists in this field, for example, often find themselves lacking in fundamental knowledge of both medicine and biology which would serve them well when choosing between headline news and material of lesser importance. There can also be disagreement on what the medical community wants to be reported, and this can have considerable ethical implications.

INCREASING MEDIA FOCUS ON MEDICINE

'The question is no longer whether physicians will cooperate with the press, but when, how and to what degree they will cooperate.'[1] William C. DeVries, who made this remark, had a notable medical first when, in December 1982, he implanted an artificial heart into one of his patients, Barney C. Clark. This operation attracted impressive news coverage as did a second similar one. The public could, as it were, witness at first hand the patient's agony, and the surgeon and his team reaped the benefit of the publicity. It is surely beyond doubt today that the medical community cannot deny the existence of a press which gets daily increasingly curious about the advances of medicine and its occasional mistakes. Refusal to cooperate with the media is useless. The news will get out in any case through another and possibly less well-informed source. There are many reasons for this situation. Perhaps most importantly, there is a real and growing public demand. Health has become a genuine and major concern for every one of us. Life expectation is better and the accent has moved from illness and disease to a more positive approach. The growing number of television chat shows on medical subjects as diverse as the herpes virus and breast surgery, testifies to the demand. In response to this, the media, whether in the form of print, television, or radio, set aside more space each day for medical or health-related topics. The press can go as far as devoting more than a third of a publication to health articles as shown by Hicks in her study of the content of daily newspapers.[2] The media interest can also be explained partly by the fact that those who control the media are just as interested in health. If an editor-in-chief needs to undergo an examination or follow a special diet, or if his son has received poor treatment, or his wife is having problems caused by her birth-control pills, it is likely he will ask one of his reporters to investigate that particular topic. There is thus a double demand—demand from the public which the press claims to know from volume of correspondence received, and demand from the press chiefs themselves, often arising from their domestic or dinner-party experiences! The so-called public demand tends to increase too. The phrase 'our readers have a right to know' is open to many interpretations. Events can be largely created where there was originally very little to say. And unfortunately, real public health issues can be ignored because elements in the hierarchy have no particular interest or regard the matter as dull or taboo. Thus quantities of air-time and print are spent discussing the spread of the human immunodeficiency virus (HIV), while teenage pregnancy, tuberculosis, pneumococcus-induced pneumonia, and incontinence in the elderly are largely ignored.[3] Rare but spectacular surgical feats, such as multiple transplants or the separation of Siamese twins, will always find room in the press and on television. Health has now become a real arena for media competition.

RESPONSIBILITY IN MEDICAL REPORTING

This explosion of medical news has led the press to use reporters capable of breaking down the professional barriers and coming up with information that will sell before their competitors get a chance to do so. This increase in the number of medical correspondents or reporters has happened without the requirement of any training or specialized knowledge in the field.

To understand the difficulties such reporters can encounter, we need only recall the recent Nobel prizes awarded to specialists in molecular biology. Without some knowledge of medicine or biology, or access to reliable sources, it is impossible to explain satisfactorily monoclonal antibodies or growth factors, or even the rearrangement of nucleic acids in the antibody coding. All too often medical journalists lack the necessary background to understand fully the contents of a written press release. In considering a new kind of treatment, for example, one of the most basic precautions is to refer to the clinical papers in reputable scientific journals before proclaiming it as a miracle. But these are often not available at short notice to a busy reporter fighting to meet a deadline. The news comes in from agency dispatches and is often released without consulting the original documents.[4]

This state of affairs is being increasingly exploited by the pharmaceutical industry which takes advantage of journalists' deficiencies as much as possible. Thus, in countries where drugs restricted to medical prescription cannot be advertised publicly, press conferences tend to be held where the product is presented more or less officially. After the conference, a reporter may write an article about it which is eventually read by hundreds of thousands of people, cut out of the newspapers, and subsequently found in doctors' waiting rooms where the product is demanded as *the* treatment by substantial numbers of patients. In France in 1988 a popular publication and a tabloid newspaper published a report on the possible cure of hypertension using a calcium inhibitor. This was in fact nothing more than a longer-lasting version of an established medicine, verapamil. It was then left to the doctors to explain as best they could to their hypertensive patients that this revolutionary cure was no more than a clever marketing stunt.

This is unfortunately not an isolated example. There was a similar story in the United States with the anti-hypertensive drug Minoxidil, which ended up becoming a treatment for baldness. The Food and Drug Administration (FDA), dissatisfied with the manufacturer's instructions, refused to endorse its sale, but Americans soon discovered that it was readily available in both Canada and Mexico. The same dubious honours have been given by the press to other so-called miracle products, such as Ribavarine or AL-721,[5] while the health authorities were simultaneously rejecting them as treatments for AIDS. These products nevertheless benefited from widespread publicity through articles which lacked in research and accuracy written in a field where everyone wants to find a good story and write it before a rival. The medical scoop is the shared obsession of the media, and to achieve it they often ignore or violate official sanctions and caveats and report new techniques before they have been properly and scientifically evaluated.[6]

THE BOUNDARIES OF TRUTH

A few years ago, Jay Winsten[7] asked 20 top American journalists a series of questions about their working methods and particular difficulties. They all agreed that the need to make the front page was what caused them most anguish on a daily basis and that their editors were the force behind this. As one of them put it, such pressure forced them to go 'right up to the boundaries of truth'—to sell a story to an editor, it was necessary to embellish it in such a way that it became clear that they were straying from the strict facts.

This need to go too far is the result of both internal and external conflict—the journalist needs to be regarded as the paper's medical expert while at the same time beat rival journalists to the finishing line. The editor tends to rely on his expert to provide him with medical material and does not himself have the knowledge to assess the quality of that material. Indeed a better informed and more responsible journalist in this field may suffer by refusing to develop what seems to be a story of minor interest and importance when competing publications, unashamed of their lack of integrity, exploit and expand the details to make a story where none exists. Going beyond the boundaries of truth then is a constant threat in medical journalism—the dilemma is how to preserve both journalistic and scientific integrity.

Even major newspapers are not exempt from criticism of their treatment of medical matters. The case of Baby Jane Doe is one example of this. Baby Doe was born in October 1983 in Uniondale, New York, suffering from multiple anomalies including spina bifida and microcephaly. Without surgery she was bound to die and even with it, severe and permanent handicaps would remain. A heated debate followed, fuelled largely by the local and international media, as to whether the baby should be allowed to live or not. With reference to specific articles, Klaidman and Beauchamp,[8] delivered a stern rebuke to such major titles as the *New York Times*, the *Los Angeles Times*, and the *Washington Post*. Many of their 'facts' on the baby's condition had not been taken from medical sources. They reported that she was lacking a large part of the brain, particularly that which controls learning faculties, while describing her as leaping on to her father's lap and smiling at him. Legal, philosophical, and even medical questions were left unanswered. The parents' decision to refuse all surgery and the administration's stance against their refusal were hardly mentioned. But most astonishing of all was the fact that only a handful of medical correspondents were assigned to the story. It was seen as predominantly a human interest rather than a medical story and reporters with no scientific background whatsoever were assigned to cover it. The decision was taken to sell the story rather than to approach it from a more scientific standpoint and examine the serious ethical and human questions which arise from the progress of medicine and biotechnology.

CONFLICT BETWEEN PRODUCTION AND CONSUMPTION OF MEDICAL KNOWLEDGE

This sadly is by no means the only example of the conflict between the production and consumption of scientific knowledge, essentially a conflict in which accuracy, pressure for speedy publication, and profit are all involved. Words such as cancer, cholesterol, and AIDS in bold headlines are guaranteed to rocket the sales of newspapers. This is another illustration of the conflict of interests in this field— the interests of the pharmaceutical and biotechnological companies and their advertising agencies, the newspapers and television stations and their competitors.

One of the most common tactics used by companies and agencies is to make a journalist believe he is being singled out for preferential treatment when an important piece of news—such as a new method of identifying heart disease or rapid detection of anti-HIV antibodies—is entrusted only to him. The idea is to release the story at the end of the week, preferably late on a Friday night—in enough detail to warrant further enquiry. This makes it difficult for the journalist to find anyone to consult during the weekend either from the company concerned or from his regular professional sources. He is reluctant not to publish anything on Monday and risk having a competitor get the story out before him. Even an incorrect or incomplete version would still be the *first* report and he knows he could not justify to his editor failure to publish at least what he had. The story can be corrected in later versions but by then the essential aim of the public relations companies has been achieved. These practices have proliferated since the development of biotechnological companies and their representation in the financial markets. Their shares increase on the strength of the 'news' and they collect their rewards and slip swiftly out of the limelight as the story fades away.

Situations such as these, however, do not only originate as a result of the activities of profit-hungry companies—sometimes they can benefit without any personal involvement. In 1985, for example, the French Government, at the instigation of the then Minister of Health, Georgina Dufoix, announced astonishing results achieved through the use of Ciclosporine in treating AIDS. A press conference was called and nine of the patients under treatment were introduced.[9] A few days later the whole affair faded away when two of the patients died. But meanwhile Sandoz, the manufacturer of the drug, while not being responsible for the story, had benefited from an increase of more than 10% in its assets on the Zurich stock market.

DANGERS OF OVER-SIMPLIFICATION AND CHANGE OF EMPHASIS

If the press in general leaves much to be desired, it must also be said that seemingly reputable sources are often guilty of inaccuracy or over-simplification also. There are scientific magazines which aim to inform the general public and these are often used as reference sources by medical journalists. These publications have a tendency to simplify the contents of papers from medical journals,[10] using summaries and abstracts embellished with provocative titles which do not always reflect reality. Adams Smith,[11] for example, describes how the British magazine the *New Scientist* rewrote a scientific paper from the medical weekly *The Lancet*.

In its issue of 2 June 1984, *The Lancet* published the results of a study by Canadian workers in a group of 40 Filipino betel chewers. Betel is suspected of being carcinogenic, and oral cancer is frequent in Asia. The Filipino study group had their diet supplemented for three months with capsules of beta-carotence and retinol. Cells were then scraped from inside their cheeks in order to evaluate the frequency of cells with micronuclei, a phenomenon reflecting chromosome breakage and increased by carcinogenic stimuli. On completion of the trial, the researchers noted simply that supplementation was associated with a three-fold decrease in the mean proportion of cells with micronuclei.

Rewritten by the *New Scientist* the emphasis changed. 'Extra vitamin A could help protect the millions of Asians who chew betel quid every day from getting mouth cancer...Giving regular quid chewers capsules of vitamin A and pro-vitamin A can reduce the number of abnormal cheek cells by more than 75%...' There is no room here for hesitation or equivocation. The results are not 'suggesting the possibility that' but become 'the authors discovered...' What was suggested as a possible association in the original *Lancet* article has become a direct cause–effect relationship in the *New Scientist*.

Such amendments to the original are found in magazines whose main purpose is to decode scientific languague for an intelligent lay readership generally composed of teachers and students.[12] And they are dangerous because such readers hold positions of discursive authority in their respective communities. Once health issues have been inaccurately reported, particularly in a 'respectable' scientific journal, it is difficult for the medical community to re-establish the truth. It is unfortunate that magazines whose titles include the word science or one of its derivatives are not more meticulous in the treatment of the articles they offer their readership.

Like any other consumer, doctors must not compromise themselves to an all-powerful press.[12] They should speak out when incorrect information is given or when an article's content is questionable and could lead to general misunderstanding and further problems for the medical community. It is imperative that they warn journalists when such situations arise. It is their professional duty to advise a publication or network that no further cooperation will be forthcoming if mistakes persist and, should their request be ignored, to instigate legal action to ensure clarification of a given point. We cannot justify absolute medical power, but it would be equally outrageous to allow inaccurate and misleading information on health matters to go unchallenged. Everyone would benefit from a situation where rules were more clearly defined and mistakes rectified.

ROLE OF MEDICAL INSTITUTIONS IN JOURNALISM

Among other sources which can influence the work of medical journalists are of course the hospitals and medical institutions themselves. Hospitals, public or private, are no longer the distant sanctuaries they once were. They have become fertile ground for investigative journalism, a fact which most of them accept to a greater or lesser extent. Many of them have now set up their own press offices.

Some hospitals and other medical institutions refuse this type of cooperation. This is criticized by DeVries[1] on the grounds that a journalist will say or write something anyway to satisfy his editor, and, without well-informed input from health professionals, more mistakes will be made. There is also the danger that, deprived of comment from the hospital, reporters will make commercial overtures to the patients and their relatives direct, often with considerable financial inducement to obtain exclusive coverage. In this situation anything goes—including even a patient's permission to be photographed, either by a family member of even by a reporter using a hidden camera. In this way, information about new techniques or questions of ethics is given by spokesmen with no medical background whatsoever who merely repeat what they can grasp of the matter, and the story is taken up again by the press with inaccurate and distorted results.

If some hospitals are excessively cautious and reticent, however, there are also at the other extreme those which are over-enthusiastic and confuse the task of informing with that of public relations. This was shown in a study by Hicks and Flint,[13] about the recriminations of journalists in the face of particular hospital managers who summoned them to show off a specific medical or surgical achievement expecting only wide and uncritical coverage.[14] If the journalists had questions to ask, however, or if discussion took an unexpected turn, there was seldom a staff member available for comment.

This approach too can only damage the quality of information released to the public. In attempting to show only the bright side and avoid discussion of the economic and other implications of any procedure, the press is reduced to a purely promotional role on behalf of a particular hospital or procedure. This happened in Los Angeles, for example, where television station KHJ invited a plastic surgeon to describe his 'revolutionary' method of enlarging breast size through prosthesis. Attracted by the results presented in the programme, a young woman decided to undergo the operation and registered herself shortly thereafter at the surgeon's clinic. The operation failed and the woman successfully sued both the surgeon and the television station.[15] The confusion of news with public relations also puts journalists in a difficult position. If they feel they have been used in an almost humiliating way, they are bitter towards those they feel have exploited them. The converse may also occur when the insitutions genuinely need the help of the press and find instead only hostile reporters trying to find a story behind the story rather than relaying the real facts of an important public health issue.

NEED FOR ETHICAL STANDARDS AND COOPERATION

While hospitals have certainly learned how to use the media to their advantage, so have many doctors themselves increasingly understood the financial and other benefits of making themselves known. The market exists—the media need both medical news and doctors capable of explaining it. Some doctors capitalize on their expert status—no matter what their specialist field, they have much to say on all subjects. Others use their personal fame and standing to promote products while their own involvement with the product is not always made clear. In 1987 the FDA, for example, harshly criticized the manufacturer of a facial cream which claimed to achieve nothing less than complete skin regeneration.[15] One of the product's sponsors was Dr Christian Barnard, the celebrated South African surgeon who performed the first successful heart transplant in 1967.[16]

Should it be a heart surgeon's business to promote the merits of cosmetic products? The FDA seems in part to have answered this question by censuring 22 companies in the same year and demanding that their advertising strategy be changed. As for Dr Barnard, he now holds a counselling post at a Swiss clinic which specializes in regenerating skin tissue by fresh cell transplant—a technique forbidden in many countries!

From the point of view of ethics, there are many reasons for infringement of rules in regard to medical information. Even if such occurrences are relatively uncommon, their very existence emphasizes the inadequacy of those regulations designed to protect us and suggest that such regulations need to be tightened or redefined. Protective measures are becoming increasingly necessary,[17] especially where there has been a rapid expansion in local broadcasting. Regional and town-based stations are fast becoming commonplace in Europe and health is perhaps the main issue guaranteed to boost the ratings. We are therefore moving inevitably towards an increase in health material being needed at this level, with all the attendant risks and misinformation this could involve. The aim then is one of minimizing the margin of error without infringing freedom of expression. Quality news must be brought to a demanding public without promoting doctors for their own gain. This is not an easy task.

The compelling need to rethink the ethical rules becomes evident when we consider outbreaks of diseases such as AIDS where the press acts as the watchdog of public health,[18] and accordingly where economic and social concerns are involved. Should doctors then be in charge of medical news? This is surely impracticable and undesirable. Difficulties encountered in many countries could jeopardize quality by attracting inferior doctors into journalism as a method of avoiding unemployment. Doctors should of course be involved in providing medical news where specialist knowledge is needed, but those chosen must be competent and properly trained. Only by raising the standards of medical journalism itself will the problem be solved.

So the participation of the medical community is essential for the improvement of the information released. The power doctors hold gives them the right to read an article before publication or to preview a story before it is broadcast under the pretext of checking scientific precision. The media cannot refuse their request for fear of losing cooperation and with it the story itself. Roy Calne has described this as an abuse of power and states that doctors tend to be the first to obtain for themselves what they usually deny others.[19] It is unreasonable for them to condemn the press for talking of a miracle treatment while at the same time setting themselves up as arbiters of the truth. The press is not necessarily wrong simply because a doctor claims it is. Whelan and Stanko, worried about the proliferation of medical broadcasting, draw attention to the doctors' inclination to play along with the media.[20] The aim instead should be to find a position, neither hostile nor indulgent, where they could act as professionals in their field instead of media stars. Such guidelines are difficult to compose and to follow because different countries have different laws to regulate medical practice. In France, for example, the use of personalities in advertising can lead to legal proceedings while in the United States a doctor can tell us with impunity why he chose a particular make of computer. What is needed is a clear admission that the professions of medicine and journalism are very different, an understanding of those differences, and an effort to build bridges and reach a more comfortable and productive *modus vivendi* from both points of view.

NEED FOR TRAINING

Because most medical journalists are not medically qualified, it should be necessary for them to have periodic training and briefing. This would allow them to read medical papers and exercise their critical faculties with some measure of independence. It would also familiarize them with concepts such as cost-benefit and cost-effectiveness, which would help to explain the logic behind certain public health decisions and why a particular medicine should not be introduced on the grounds of excessive cost and lack of results compared to its competitors.

This training could with mutual advantage be a two-way process. Medical associations and universities could be involved, with the added advantage of journalists being exposed to quality lecturers and the institutions themselves to the profession of journalism with all its constraints and pressures.

Medical training should also include an introduction to the world of the media— how it operates, the advantages and disadvantages of working in partnership with it, and its limitations and pitfalls. This would be an asset to all doctors, especially with the developing local broadcasting networks, and it would make a greater number of qualified people and specialists available for consultation and comment.

In addition, a doctor who learned to simplify and condense his language for the benefit of an audience would himself benefit in his daily dealings with his patients and in his professional life.

CONCLUSIONS

Today, with the modification of many aspects of public health we have not only a better informed public but more specialized and complicated news. Many interests are involved—medical, social, ethical, political, and economic. Quality news depends on the recognition of all the above, and many journalists recognize this. But they need to be helped not used by their natural allies, the doctors, the pharmaceutical companies, and the administrators. Equally, the media itself must understand that it cannot act irresponsibly in the name of freedom. Open and intelligent relationships are essential if we are to have ethically sound as well as top quality medical news.

The time has surely come for all those involved in the field of health care and medicine to try to define a set of rules to encourage all concerned to work together. A good starting point might be a sensible consideration of and agreement on the use of embargo rules. This procedure, which prevents an item being released before a given day and time, should be rigorously enforced since it would put all media on an equal footing. Happily, major medical publications such as the *New England Journal of Medicine* have moved to tighten the rules in this respect.[21-24]

Ultimately, improved understanding and mutual respect between health professionals and journalists should result in a better standard of medical journalism providing sound information on health to the consumers, in this case patients. And better informed patients will be easier patients to deal with.

In the long term, this will also serve the goals of responsible and effective health education. The media are potent influences for good or ill. Used skilfully and with a proper respect for accuracy, they can ensure that everyone becomes better able to take appropriate steps towards positive health and the avoidance of disease. In an ideal world the medical journalist could become a powerful ally of all those involved in health education.[25]

REFERENCES

1. DeVries, W. The physician, the media, and the 'spectacular' case. *J Am Med Assoc* 1988; **259(6)**: 886–890.
2. Hicks, N. 1986 newspaper survey by Hill and Knowlton hospital marketing and communication service. *Hospitals* 1986; **60**: 6.
3. Flaysakier, W. Television, radio, et santé. *Concourse Med* 1988; **110(2)**: 134.
4. Hicks, N. Public health, public policy and 'neon' issues in ethics. *Med J Aust* 1985; **143**: 104–107.
5. Barinaga, M. Controversial AIDS drug for US market. *Nature* 1988; **332**: 475.

6. Gunby, P. Media-abetted liver transplants raise questions of 'equity and decency'. *J Am Med Assoc* 1983; **249(15)**: 1973–74, 1980–1.
7. Winsten, J. Science and the Media: the boundaries of Truth. *Hlth Affairs* 1985; **4(1)**: 5–23.
8. Klaidman, S. and Beauchamp, T.L. Baby Jane Doe in the media. *J Hlth Politics Policy Law* 1986; **11(2)**. 271–284.
9. Agence France Presse. La ciclosporine dans le traitement du sida. October 29, 1985.
10. Leese, H.J. Communicating science to the public (Letter to the Editor). *Human Reprod* 1986; **1(7)**: 495.
11. Adams Smith, D.E. The process of popularization—rewriting medical research papers for the layman: discussion paper. *J R Soc Med* 1987; **80**: 634–636.
12. Lesse, S. Research perormed under the mass-media stage. Questions of reliability and ethics. *Am J Psychother* 1985; **39(1)**: 1–3.
13. Hicks, N. and Flint, J. Ceos and the media strive for balance. *Hospitals* 1988; 5 March: 42–44.
14. Friedman, E. What's eroding hospital's image? *Hospitals* 1985; 15 September; 76, 79–82.
15. *Le Monde*. Diafoirus de l'information. July 6 1988.
16. *Advertising Age*. Ten categories that will make news in '88. p. 2. December 28, 1987.
17. Rene, L. Medias et deontologie. *Bull Acad Ntle Med* 1987; **171**: 6725–6732.
18. Check, W. Public education on AIDS: not only the media's responsibility. *Hastings Center Report*. Special Supplement 1985; **15(4)**: 27–31.
19. Calne, R. Medicine and the media. *Br Med J* 1988; **206**: 1389.
20. Whelan, E.M. and Stanko, R.T. Medically muddled media. *J Am Med Assoc* 1983; **250**: 2137.
21. Relman, A.S. The Ingelfinger Rule. *N Engl J Med* 1981; **305**: 824–26.
22. Relman, A.S. More on the Ingelfinger Rule. *N Engl J Med* 1988; **318**: 1125–1126.
23. The Steering Committee of the Physicians' Health Study Group. Preliminary Report. *N Engl J Med* 1988; **318**: 262.
24. Altman, L.K. Medical guardians. *New York Times* **1988**, 28 January 1988.
25. Nau, J.Y. Informations à caractère médical dans la presse écrite d'audience nationale. Education sanitarie ou journalisme? Thèse pour le Doctorat en Médecine 1984. Faculté de Médecine de Tours, France.

SECTION III

TARGET GROUPS

CHAPTER 8

Ethics of Health Education for Children

SPYROS DOXIADIS AND TINA GARANIS

'In children may be observed the traces and seeds of what will one day be settled
psychological habits.'

(Aristotle)

SUMMARY

Ethical problems of health education with respect to young children exist even
during their infancy and childhood. They arise from the unconscious absorption
by them of sometimes intended but mainly unintended messages derived from
their family environment, preschool education, and television. These sources,
constituting a hidden curriculum, influence to a great extent their knowledge and
later attitudes and behaviour. After a brief description of their learning abilities
until they reach school age, the various types of influences from their environment
are described. A discussion follows of the important issue of children's rights and
autonomy in relation to their parents' obligations. We end with recommendations
addressed to parents, professionals, and those responsible for mass communication
media.

INTRODUCTION

It is now generally recognized and accepted that children are able to learn and
imitate actions from as early as the neonatal period. It is, therefore, reasonable
to conclude and necessary to accept that messages which have some relation to
health habits and lifestyles will influence the infant's and young child's behaviour.
Furthermore, they will form a foundation on which their knowledge, attitudes, and
behaviour for the rest of their lives will be based.

Since the ethical problems of health education in schools are covered by Downie
and Fyfe in the next chapter, we will deal here with the age period from infancy to

Ethics in Health Education
Edited by S. Doxiadis. ©1990 John Wiley & Sons Ltd

school entry, which in most countries takes place at 5 to 6 years of age. However, most of what we have to say about influences operating at home and generally outside school applies equally to school-age children.

In the first years of life most of what children learn is unconsciously absorbed by them from the people around them. Whether we try to or not, whether we like it or not, our acts and words influence them. We cannot avoid it. Young children gain much of their learning from direct experience of people and events.

Thus it is useful to begin with a brief description of the stages of development of learning ability during the first years of life and then proceed to examine all factors in the environment which leave their imprint on the child. Next we shall examine the ethical and legal basis of parents' authority over their children. The main part of the chapter will concentrate on the ethical issues arising in the field of wanted or unwanted, conscious or unconscious, health education of young children. We shall conclude with some suggestions and recommendations for all those responsible for young children—parents, caretakers, nursery school teachers, and all other individuals, such as those working in the mass communication media, whose activities are likely to send information and messages to children.

STAGES OF DEVELOPMENT

We mentioned at the beginning of this chapter that learning begins even at the neonatal period. This is clear from the observation that young infants mimic the actions of those facing them, such as putting out their tongue. This may appear of no importance because it does not show any more longlasting effects, it does not demonstrate any more general influence on present and future behaviour.

There are, however, studies of the last 50 years showing the deep and longlasting effects of experiences and events occurring in infancy and early childhood, not only in the cognitive field, but also—more importantly—in personality development. The works of Spitz,[1] Anna Freud,[2] Bowlby,[3] and many others since, have shown that early environmental circumstances, such as absence of adequate sensory stimulation and deprivation of maternal love, have longlasting and even permanent effects on the development of cognitive ability, temperament, and personality.

Let us now review briefly the stages of development regarding mainly the field of learning. Since in the first two to three years of life the child does not have the verbal abilities to express clearly what he has learnt or understood, we have to gather information from the observable development in the field of hearing and language on the one hand, and of social behaviour on the other. Here very briefly are some milestones relevant to the young child's ability to understand, recognize, and act accordingly. At 12–18 months of age he understands simple commands and although he may play alone he needs an adult nearby. At 18–24 months he carries out verbal requests, mimics domestic acts, and responds to adult guidance. At 2–3 years he repeats and sings nursery rhymes, uses language for questioning, and begins to help with dressing and undressing. He also helps with tidying away.

At 3–4 years he can understand and repeat long stories and begins imaginative play in which children play adult roles. Everyday activities are imitated and he is able to understand good and bad. Finally, at 4–5 years he can speak fluently, and he has become more independent and confident. His play is influenced by his sex and his environment and therefore by the culture to which he belongs.

Throughout all these stages of development there is continuous and continuing integration of various activities. Each new skill and attainment is the result of the development of the appropriate receptive channels, and it appears at the most appropriate time so that use is made of any messages and information received.

The advantages of such integration, as summarized by Holt,[4] are the following:

(a) Developmental integration increases the scope of any one of the receptive channels by linking it with other receptive channels, and effectiveness of any action is increased by links with other means of expressive response.
(b) Developmental integration increases the potential for learning and for effective action.
(c) Developmental integration promotes the smoothness of the developmental pattern.
(d) Developmental integration creates a possibility of utilizing alternative means for acquiring information and carrying out actions. The possession of alternative means to achieve a particular goal is biologically most important, because if one route is blocked then compensatory mechanisms can be evoked. The importance of this is seen in the case of many handicapped children.

These integrative processes also make clear the close link between incoming messages through the receptive channels and the ensuing acts.

All the progress and developmental changes described above come about as a result of interacting with other people. But a note of caution must be sounded here, especially addressed to readers not familiar with the discipline of child development. What makes each one of us be what we are and behave as we behave, is the product of a continuous interaction of our genetic endowment with the influences of our environment, including the intrauterine. For description, analysis, and discussion of this vast topic the reader is referred to the recent book *Early Influences Shaping the Individual*.[5]

For the purpose of the present chapter it is sufficient to say that, no matter what the genetic make-up of a child is, the experiences and messages received from his environment influence his knowledge, his attitudes, and his behaviour from the first weeks of life. This process of socialization should be understood as the result of a social interaction between the parents—or other caretakers—and the child. As Schaffer[6] very clearly explains:

'...the study of parental control techniques shows clearly that the demands a parent makes on a child are every bit as much a function of the child's state and behaviour at the time as of the parent's requirements; socialization, that is, cannot be understood merely by looking at the parent but must be considered as an interactional activity.'

WHAT IS 'ENVIRONMENT' FOR THE PRESCHOOL CHILD?

The answer to this question would have been very simple until a few decades ago. Then almost all influences operating on the child during the first five or six years of his life were from the nuclear family or extended family. This is not now the case. In all developed countries and perhaps in many of the developing countries, the small child receives messages sent intentionally or unintentionally from a variety of sources. It is not only that many more persons come into contact with him, such as individual caretakers or the staff of day care facilities and nursery schools. It is also the presence of the all-pervading mass communication media, almost exclusively television, because preschool children do not read and seldom understand the spoken word from radio. The third source of information and messages, hidden or not, is the nursery school.

Since the ethics of health education in schools are discussed in the next chapter, we shall concentrate here mainly on influences from the family, from television, and from other caretaker groups. All send messages to young children in different ways, through actions and words and we will, therefore, examine them separately.

Influences from the Family

The actions and words of the people around small children, usually parents and siblings, other relatives and less often other unrelated persons such as all sorts of caretakers, give continuous messages to them. They acquire knowledge, which forms attitudes, which result in certain types of behaviour. The messages given are often unintentional—the hidden curriculum—or they aim specifically at forming a desired type of behaviour. Examples follow of the various day-to-day activities going on in the home and closely related to health, lifestyle, and hence health education.

(a) *Nutrition*. It is likely that breast feeding with the close proximity of mother and baby and the sense of satisfaction given to the mother, has some positive psychological effects on the infant. The beneficial effects of breast feeding on the physical health of the infant are generally accepted but the likely influence on mental health is not proven. Nutrition and feeding habits after the first year of life, however, exert long-surviving influences. Obese babies and small children are more likely to become obese adolescents and adults. Recent work has shown that the damage to heart and vessels which manifests later in life may have its origin during infancy and childhood.[7] In addition to the physical effects, the habit of overeating, of eating too many sweets, of snacking between meals, can very well be established in the preschool years. Related to this also are habits of oral hygiene, that is regular mouthwashing and brushing of teeth which, mimicking adults and encouraged by them, should start in early childhood.

(b) *Alcohol consumption* in the family is another potent message given to small children. If strong drinks are regularly consumed by the adult members of the family, if beer and wine are always present at meals the message is given that alcohol forms a normal part of daily life. The message is stronger if obvious pleasure is shown by the drinking adult. A different kind of message is given if any person in the family is seen in a drunken state. This may provoke feelings negative to alcohol.

(c) *Smoking* is another health-related message given by family members. The deleterious effects of smoking on the health of the developing organism are many and well-known: lower birthweight, higher perinatal and early infantile mortality, higher incidence of respiratory infections in the first few years of life, and finally, and perhaps more important, a small but statistically significant lowering of reading and arithmetic ability as late as the age of 10 years. But equally or more serious are the messages received that smoking is an accepted and regular habit. In their tendency to imitate adult behaviour, young children can be seen pretending to smoke using various objects such as pencils, for cigarettes.

(d) *Taking of medicines* is nowadays common in many families. Young children get used to the idea that this is a normal and regular event. Furthermore, if the mother tends to resort to medication for her children even at the first slight discomfort of a 'cold' or headache or other complaint, the idea takes root in the small child's mind that for every ill in life the remedy is a tablet or a syrup. And one can easily understand what such an attitude means when in adolescence the boy or girl meets any difficulty. The remedy for all evils that comes to their mind is drugs.

(e) Related to giving medicines is the parents' attitudes and behaviour towards doctors and other health professionals. Both extremes give negative messages. Continuous dependence on doctors by visits and telephone calls or distrust and avoidance of contact with any medical facilities may create unhealthy attitudes. Taking a sick child to the doctor and taking a healthy child for immunization are both unpleasant experiences. Even more unpleasant is admission to hospital. Proper explanation for the need for such unpleasant experiences should be given in advance. The practice in some cultures to threaten children with the doctor—'eat your food' or 'be quiet or else I'll take you to the doctor' are clearly unacceptable messages. But this is not obvious to many parents.

(f) Exercise in any form is closely linked to lifestyles directly influencing health. If small children see their parents using the car to drive a few hundred yards to work or shopping instead of walking, they will understand that the usual way to move is not on our legs but on wheels. If, on the other hand, the whole family goes for walks at weekends and appears to enjoy any king of physical exercise the message is positive; walk or other exercise is a pleasurable activity. This, as well as the following activities and aspects, work in an even more general and hidden way to influence small children.

(g) Since accidents at home and on the roads are one of the main causes of death in childhood, the behaviour of parents in this field is very important for avoidance of risks by young children. Keeping matches and medicines locked away or in special containers is a measure more of direct prevention and not so much of education. However, the correct behaviour of parents as pedestrians when accompanied by small children is essential in teaching them elementary road safety precautions.

(h) Another practical day-to-day habit is personal cleanliness. Although this may appear self-evident in developed countries it is not so in others. The habit of washing body and clothes, within the limits of each family's facilities, starts in childhood and may continue one way or other throughout life.

(i) In an even more general way, we may consider that other acts regarding the environment, such as indifference to pollution either from badly serviced cars or merely by discarding litter, make the child indifferent to the effect of the environment on mental or physical health.

(j) Attitudes to sex also have their roots early in life. If the parents give the impression that anything to do with sex—nakedness, exposing the genitalia, even questions around this topic—are sinful, the impression is gained that this is a taboo subject, and any discussion now or any later activity is something abnormal and to be condemned. Thus some later difficulties or deviations in the sex life of the adolescent and the adult may begin in childhood.

(k) Finally, since the quality of life in general is directly related to many acts affecting health, attitudes to health and healthy or unhealthy behaviour, we cannot omit acts of physical or sexual abuse and neglect. This phenomenon, existing since antiquity in many cultures, has been scientifically studied only in the last 30 years. We know now that one of the factors leading parents and other adults to abuse children is if they themselves were abused in their youth. This is the last striking example of how experiences early in life influence adult behaviour.

So what does all this amount to? Simply that knowledge and concepts about health, as well as lifestyles and behaviour affecting health, often have their roots in the influence of the environment in the early years of life. This environment is in most cases the family. Hence the duties and responsibilities of the parents which will be described in another part of this chapter.

Influences from Television

The new factor which influences children's knowledge, attitudes, and behaviour is television. In the developed countries almost all homes possess at least one set. In many homes the set is constantly on, even if no one is watching. These findings from a recent study in one of the previously most undeveloped parts of Greece confirm the results of surveys in other countries. Regular television watching extends to the preschool age. Thus 3-year-old American children were found to view television daily for an average of two and a half hours.[8]

The question arises as to what is the understanding of young children of the programmes aimed at them? Obviously this will vary according to the content of the programme, the age of the children, and their previous knowledge of the subject.[9] This is again influenced by the social and educational status of the family. Thus even in this respect children of poor and uneducated parents are disadvantaged. It has been shown that if adults are present to comment on a programme this helps understanding.[10] It has also been demonstrated that if a programme contains messages about desired types of social behaviour, preschool children absorb them and extend their learning to other situations.[11] These few examples from published work refer to viewing of programmes specially planned for young children.

There is, however, another influence: the usually unconscious absorption of messages from all kinds of programmes including advertisements, not specifically addressed to children. This is more difficult to study and assess since audience research is not possible for this age group. It is nevertheless reasonable to conclude that, as with the 'hidden' curriculum from contacts with living individuals, exposure to casual and unintentional television viewing leaves traces in young children's minds with often unpredictable effects on their behaviour.

The observations and results described above are only a small sample of the many works on the influence of television on children. This topic is fully reviewed in an extensive publication from the United States National Institutes of Mental Health.[12]

Finally, Postman in his book *The Disappearance of Childhood: How TV is Changing Children's Lives* goes as far as to claim that the influence of extensive television viewing abolishes the boundaries separating childhood from adulthood and thus destroys the normal and necessary process of physiological maturation.[13]

Other Caretaker Groups

The growing population of working mothers and one parent families has in the last 20 years considerably increased the number of infants and young children who spend some hours every day in an environment outside their home, whether in kindergartens, nursery or infant schools or other day-care facilities. They are, therefore, influenced by the teaching and general behaviour of all those working in these environments, be they trained personnel or other workers, such as volunteers or cleaners.

Much of what is said in the next chapter for school teachers applies to the trained caretakers and their responsibilities as well. As far as the other individuals are concerned, their behaviour in matters of health habits (smoking, cleanliness, pollution) may have the same type of influence as the behaviour of those at home. This influence is weaker, however, because of a more limited exposure of infants and young children to the presence and to the acts of these individuals.

We may state as a general conclusion that infants and young children absorb information and messages from many sources, the main ones being home environment, television, and preschool day-care facilities. Their attitudes and acts are shaped accordingly. We have to realize that anything that happens in their environment from early infancy onwards is likely to be part of their health education.

The effects on their actions of these early influences are difficult to assess because a large part of their daily life is regulated by their parents. Parents prepare the food, remind the children to wash their hands, to brush their teeth; they restrict eating of snacks and sweets between meals. Young children at home have no chance of really independent action; and if they have, it is difficult for the outside observer to separate what they do spontaneously and what under the prompting of their parents.

Their behaviour during late childhood, adolescence, and adulthood, is again influenced by many factors, operating after they enter school. Teachers, peers, television, cinema all contribute. It is not therefore possible to attribute unequivocally a certain lifestyle or a certain health habit at the age of 15 or 20 years or later to preschool influences.

There have been attempts to study children's views of health[14] or their attitudes, for example, toward thinness and fatness,[15] but these are not relevant to our subject. We are left, therefore, with the results of other studies mentioned previously which have generally shown that both knowledge and attitudes shaping later behaviour have their origins in the first years of life. And on this general conclusion we must base what will follow. Before we go into the ethical implications of this statement, however, we should examine the rights and responsibilities of parents and children from a philosophical and from a legal point of view.

CHILDREN AND AUTONOMY

Joseph Goldstein wrote

'To be a *child* is to be at risk, dependent and without capacity or authority to decide what is best for oneself. To be an *adult* is to be a risktaker, independent and with capacity and authority 'to decide what is "best" for oneself. To be an *adult who is a parent* is to be presumed in law to have the capacity, authority and responsibility to determine and to do what is good for one's children.'[16]

Parental responsibilities which begin as early as conception, are, according to the Council of Europe,[17] a collection of duties and powers which aim at ensuring the moral and material welfare of the child by providing mainly for his education and his maintenance. It is not difficult to see why health care and health education are a vital part of these responsibilities: every person lives in his body and every person *is* his body in a certain sense. A child, in particular, grows up in his body for this body is the shell in which his development takes place. Therefore, his physical and mental health are of major importance.

We shall deal in this part with the philosophical justification of parental authority over a child's health care and education and we shall also refer briefly to the position of this authority in the various legal systems. In the next part of the chapter we shall deal with the ethical implications which derive from the exercising of such an authority.

The justification of parental authority is based on the recognition of the fact that small children are unable to take proper care of themselves; therefore, somebody else must take care of them. And children cannot take care of themselves because they lack autonomy, that is the capacity to think rationally and decide by choosing a certain course of action in the absence of various constraints. Thus, a person is autonomous only if these conditions are satisfied.

Deciding whether a person is autonomous or not involves a complex moral argumentation for people to agree that lack of autonomy justifies a paternalistic attitude. What they disagree with is the *description* of a particular case: others may describe the same person as non-autonomous because they use a different set of criteria or the same criteria applied to a different degree. This problem, however, does not arise in the case of very young children; on the contrary, these children are considered to be typical examples of non-autonomous agents, unable to make the appropriate decisions.

Normally it is the parents, as we have already seen, who must decide on their child's behalf. The obligation to decide on behalf of somebody else poses an immense burden of responsibility on the proxy's shoulders. The obligation to decide for a child, however, is even more difficult, for children possess a certain characteristic which other non-autonomous agents lack: this characteristic is the potentiality to develop—under normal circumstances—to future fully autonomous agents. We do not wish to imply that in other cases—for example, in the case of a mentally handicapped person—the decision-maker should feel less responsible because of the possible futility of the case. Yet it is difficult to deny that when we speak about children we often think of what lies ahead, of the grown-ups that these children will one day become. The notion of childhood involves the notion of the future and everything that has a future acquires a greater importance in our minds. This is quite justifiable in the case of children; it is the negative consequences deriving from such a way of thinking that are unjustifiable—that is, neglecting those persons who do *not* have a future ahead. It is true that, when the question of autonomy is discussed, children are referred to in parallel with the mentally ill, mentally handicapped, or senile people. But is is also true that the degree of interest is not the same in each one of these examples, for all these groups of persons are being taken care of in a completely different way and the aim of this care varies from a better use of the person's potential in the case of children to a simple—and not always a dignified—survival in the case of the senile.

Let us, however, return to our starting point, that paternalism in health care is justified because children are not autonomous agents. Moreover, children are unable to grasp the notion of health, and the more holistic this notion becomes the more difficult it is for everybody, and not only children, to understand. Most adults are usually in a position to know—even roughly—how their body functions. Children are not in this position because they lack the knowledge they need in order to grasp the difference between what healthy and unhealthy means.

A young child is able to understand only the empirical facts. He may know, for example, that eating too much ice cream might make him sick. What he does not know is why this happens. A child is able to express his wishes; he knows empirically that he prefers some tastes to some others. But young children do not know anything about vitamins or proteins and they cannot realise the importance of good and bad nutritional habits. They are able to decide according to their taste; but they are unable to perform the balancing of risks and benefits that decisions about their health require, because this mechanism of thought is too complex for them.

Children lack autonomy because autonomy does not require only the mere, empirical knowledge of some facts. It also requires a careful deliberation of these facts and the decision to follow a particular course of action. Children can fulfil the first requirement; they cannot fulfil the second. This distinction was clearly expressed by J.S. Mill when he said about individual sovereignty over one's own mind and body:

'it is perhaps hardly necessary to say that this doctrine is meant to apply only to human beings in the maturity of their faculties. We are not speaking of children or of young persons below the age which the law may fix as that of manhood or womanhood. Those who are still in a state to require being taken care of by others, must be protected against their own actions as well as against external injury.'[18]

Parental responsibilities are imposed and recognized by most legal systems. The argument goes as follows: since children are unable to take care of themselves somebody else must do that. The most appropriate people are the child's parents because the sincerity of good parental intentions and the existence of genuine concern are taken for granted and accepted as the norm. This argument acknowledges that, in general, parents are capable of making health care choices for their children. As Anna Freud and colleagues point out,[19] where the question involves a life or death choice the state can interfere if there is sufficient evidence that parents are neglecting their parental responsibilities. If, however, the choice concerns only a preference for one lifestyle over another, the privacy of the family is generally respected. The law in many countries recognizes the right of the parents to bring up their children in the way they think is best, and this includes direct and indirect health education as well. Yet, this freedom is not an absolute one and, even when a question of lifestyle is concerned, limits of parental authority are still imposed sometimes by the law. All children, for example, are obliged by law to attend school until they reach a certain age even if their parents are of a different opinion. It is only extremely rarely that parents are allowed to educate their children solely at home and these exceptional cases not only require special permission by the educational authorities but frequent evaluation as well.

The general recognition of parental authority proves how much our society values the idea of the family. The concept of parental authority sounds very plausible and justified when very young children are concerned, for their capacity to understand and evaluate the consequences of their actions is limited. Thus, under the law, children are presumed incompetent in most domains of their life because they lack this important element of competence: the ability to reason about and appreciate the outcome of their decisions. As children grow older, however, the case of competence and autonomy becomes more and more controversial and age limits cease to be so clear-cut; although in most legal systems 18 is the year of acknowledged competence, there are wide variations from one country to another. There are also differences regarding the various fields of competence.

In past centuries children were considered to be no more than 'little people'. Now it is more and more widely recognized that children have their own nature, their own needs, and their own rights and, although the idea of children being the property of their parents has not yet completely disappeared, the Courts tend to accept that children old and mature enough to understand what is being proposed can give their own consent. This tendency reflects a different and new way to approach competence—by reference to some notion of understanding and a certain maturity. The traditional way of approaching competence has been by reference to the status of the person; that is, by his categorization into a particular context of minor, mentally handicapped, and so on. This way, has been disputed, however, because it assumes certain facts about certain categories of people. And if we can easily assume that children are not autonomous and lack competence, it is very difficult to define the age at which this comes to an end. For the law treats in the same way a child of 9 years and a 'child' of 17 years. In the former case parental authority seems the natural thing; in the latter, parental authority has to stop being absolute for, as Lord Denning once held:

> '... the legal right of a parent to the custody of a child ends at the eighteenth birthday and even up till then it is a dwindling right which the courts will hesitate to enforce against the wishes of the child, the older he is.'[20]

ETHICAL IMPLICATIONS

In every context, educating very young children is a difficult task which, because of a child's unique nature, has many ethical implications. Health care and health education do not constitute an exception to this rule; the implications are present everywhere and should not be ignored, for everything that is being taught to children during childhood is crucial to their later development.

Very often educational problems start from the educators. An important ethical question, therefore, refers to the parents' concept of health, because all parental decisions and choices concerning child health education derive from what parents define as a healthy state or a healthy way of life. Health is a very ambiguous concept and people from different sociocultural contexts give it a different meaning according to whatever theory of health is more popular in their environment. What is considered as a healthy practice in one society might be considered unhealthy in another and—on a smaller but not less important scale—what might be considered as healthy in one family might be considered unhealthy in another, or might be simply ignored as an option. The ethical problem concerns the question of whether parents are able to override their personal beliefs about health and transmit to their children objectively good and scientifically correct messages. The binding of the feet of Chinese women is a perfect example of a very unhealthy practice derived from sociocultural traditions: in these cases the parents ignored the physical welfare of their child in order not to disobey the dominant customary rules. Indirectly, this amounts to negative health education: the parents did not act according to what really was in the interest of their child but according to what was *thought to be* good for them in the particular society, irrespective of any contrary scientific opinion.

What is also important is the concept of safety. Safety, and in particular physical safety, is a crucial factor on which parents tend to base their children's health education more than on scientific data. Parents transmit such health messages so that their children will feel fine, will not hurt themselves, will not catch a cold, will not have a stomach-ache, will not break a leg or an arm. The goal of such education is not only a healthy lifestyle but a safe one as well. The notions of health and safety are often interwoven in the parents' minds. Safety, however, is also a very subjective notion. The fact that many people like to engage in risky activities, while others find the idea frightening, proves that different values are placed on different things by different people in a different way. A parent who likes to go hang-gliding every weekend, a parent who drives a motor bike to work every day, and a parent who loves mountaineering will not approach their child's health education in the same way as a parent who prefers to spend any spare time watching television. Health education can never be value-free, for health itself is not value-free.

Another important problem is the parents' education. The justification of parental authority is, as we have already said, the existence of genuine parental love and concern. Even so, deciding about a child's health and lifestyle is neither easy nor ethically trouble-free. It is true that parents normally act according to their children's best interests but the criteria they use in order to define what is 'best' may vary. The opinion of what is best is a very subjective one and the fact that a parent believes that something is good for his child does not mean that it is actually good and medically correct. Are good intentions sufficient and do they guarantee positive results? Does benevolence always end in beneficence? We all know that unfortunately it does not, and that ends do not always justify the means. On the other hand, it would be irrational to support the view that only those who happen to have a special education in health care matters are entitled to become and to continue to be parents. The natural bond and parenthood itself are sufficient guidelines, although minimal. Some of the parents, however, may go even further: they can follow special courses or seminars about child health care, they can read special books. There exist indeed endless possibilities for those who seek to learn more about their children and the way they can best care about them. But all these options exist on a voluntary basis and not a legal one. Parenthood has never required special educational qualifications. On the contrary, it is one of the very few things in the world that almost everyone can have access to and one of the very few things independent of religion, social class, colour, or educational background.

Another ethical implication concerns the variety of health care messages addressed to very young children. Although, as we have already mentioned, the State cannot intervene directly in matters concerning nothing more than a certain lifestyle, the existence of conflicting direct messages is inevitable in the kind of society and in the century that we live in. Today children receive messages from various sources: the family, the nursery, the school, the various television programmes, and the social environment. It would be naive to believe that all these messages coincide and that the views expressed in each case support the same idea. Children in fact are constantly facing a pluralism of opinions and ideas concerning their health, a pluralism which can exist in the context of the same family as well. For example, the views of a young mother concerning the nutrition of her child may differ considerably from those of the old grandmother in the family, who insists on feeding her grandchild with chocolates or toffees especially when the mother is not at home. A 3- or 4-year-old child does not have the ability to judge correctly what is being offered to him. Thus, he is simply following and mimicking the repeated messages and, if these are contradictory, the child gets confused and his health education is being undermined. It is at this very point that children feel the need of parental guidance.

Ethical problems can also arise in all day-care facilities. There, very young children are exposed to the influence of the nursery teachers, escaping temporarily from the influence of the family environment. These nursery teachers offer continuously to the children a variety of direct and indirect messages regarding their health. Have parents—should they disagree with the content of these messages—the right to interfere and prevent their children from being exposed to them? Can they demand from the caretakers and preschool teachers a certain lifestyle and a certain behaviour? Can they criticize them? Let us consider the example of smoking in the nursery schools. Do parents have the right to demand from the nursery teachers not to smoke in the presence of the children? J.S. Mill writes: 'The only purpose for which power can be rightfully exercised over any member of a civilised community against his will is to prevent harm to others.'[18] This entails a balancing of harms and benefits. Smoking indoors is certainly out of the question. Banning smoking in the playground, however, is a more complex issue. In that case there is no direct medical harm—only an indirect one—of the negative example that the smoker presents, especially to that child who has already been told at home that smoking is a bad thing. Yet, it is difficult to ban smoking in the playground on the grounds' of indirect negative influence, firstly because children, as members of a community, constantly come face to face with people who smoke (although these people are not designated as authorities for the child) and people who do many other harmful things, and secondly, because one could also support the view that the nursery teachers who work so hard with children have the right to enjoy a cigarette in the open-air playground. A complete banning might lead to a new revolutionary kind of 'school', a school where the teachers and not the pupils hide in the toilets in order to smoke! Maybe a special room for the smokers would be the most just solution.

It must also be borne in mind, however, that the question of smoking presents important differences from one country to another. In the United States, for example, the anti-smoking campaign of the Surgeon General Everett Coop has led to the banning of smoking in many public places. Many American hospitals have designated themselves non-smoking hospitals. Many big companies refuse to hire people who smoke. In Europe smoking is still popular and in some countries like Greece no-smoking areas in restaurants and other public places do not even exist. Therefore, the question of whether smoking in the playground should be banned or not should be faced in relation to the general attitudes of the particular country. Even in those countries where at present the fight against smoking is not intensive, however, every effort should be made to intensify the anti-smoking campaign. And there is a very good reason to insist on strict rules in schools, because many habits begin in childhood and because the ill effects of passive smoking, especially for small children, are well known.

Smoking, is just one example; there exist others as well, such as nutrition. The child who is being constantly told at home that chocolates are bad for his teeth, receives a harmful message when he sees his teacher at the nursery eating a chocolate every time they go to the playground. The result would not be that harmful or confusing if the person eating the 'forbidden' chocolate were another child. In such a case the feeling caused would be mere jealousy (the implications of which are equally important but outside the scope of this chapter). The teacher, however, represents power and authority in the eyes of the child and this is exactly why ethical implications arise; for conflicting messages confuse the child when they come from two different sources of authority that the child is supposed to respect and obey. It is worth noting here that maybe the messages are not conflicting; it is very possible that the teacher has already spoken to the children about the importance of keeping their teeth clean and healthy. The case of the teacher who 'forgets' the 'lesson' five minutes after it is over is even worse for the child. These problems, however, are not only a matter of the teacher's training (for nursery teachers, unlike parents, should have some specialized education concerning health care as a part of their overall training); they are also a matter of every person's character and real interest in this very special and important occupation.

Last, but not least, come the problems caused by television. It is true that by making television the scapegoat for all—or most—of the problems concerning children's education, we often exaggerate, and somehow we also divest ourselves from a part of the responsibility. Yet it is also true that television plays an important role in children's learning.

There are two different issues here. The first concerns the ethical implications which derive from the content and the effect of advertising on television. The second issue concerns the implications deriving from scientific programmes which aim to inform and educate on matters of health. Let us first consider advertising directed to children. It is obvious that the biggest part of advertising time addressed to children concerns food products, most of which have no nutritional value, and toys. The power of television is enormous because, as children do not have the maturity to judge the truthfulness and the quality of what they are being offered, for them 'seeing is believing'. Feinbloom wrote: 'An advertisement to a child has the quality of an order, not a suggestion. The child lacks the ability to set priorities, to determine relative importance, and to reject some directions as inappropriate'.[21] The child is therefore the most vulnerable, and the ideal advertisement viewer who absorbs indiscriminately every message of which he is the target. The mass of advertisements makes the parent's task even more difficult. Parents usually try to cultivate and encourage their child's ability to judge correctly, to distinguish between what is good and what is bad, to make the right choices. But as already mentioned, absolute protection from all harmful messages is impossible, for today's family structure is very different from the ideal and perfect model. Today in many families both parents work and they do not have the time—or even the right mood—to spend time with their children, to play with them, or keep them busy with something useful. Television, therefore, is the easiest and most convenient solution. An evening in front of the electronic babysitter, as television has been described, leaves the parents free to rest and the children exposed to all sorts of influences and not only to those of advertisements. Some of the questions that the research on the effects of television advertising on children has examined are the effects of violence, of food advertising, and the effect on parent–child relations.[22] This is not surprising as children keep constantly asking their parents for this 'nice toy' that they saw being advertised on television the other day and the parents keep refusing but not always with the same strength of will as their children's!

In modern society an agent therefore exists which sends messages to children well outside the control of the parents. It is easy to say that they can switch the set off or even use a special lock for the 'on' button. This cannot be done in many families for the reasons already explained, to which unemployment should be added. For many unemployed adults television is an inexpensive way to fill their time. Neither can the parents always be with the children in order to turn the set on and off according to what is being shown. It has to be repeated here that when a parent talks with the child about the contents of the programme understanding is improved and the likely negative effects may be diminished.[10]

Under these conditions it is clear that the power of the information and of all types of messages sent through television to children of all ages is enormous. The question therefore arises who will supervise this agent and how, without imposing a strict censorship, which will create resistance not only from commercial interests, but also from well-meaning people who believe in the freedom of information.

The second issue concerns the educational role of television. As Karpf points out, the mass media have a dual role in this field: first, the coverage of interesting medical topics and second, health education.[23] The most common problem of scientific programmes is the language gap and this is intensified when the programmes are addressed to children. What must also be borne in mind is that children think and feel differently from adults. Scientific programmes are always prepared by adults and all the relevant data are presented from an adult's point of view. This may neglect the feelings of children who can easily become frightened and be falsely impressed. It is very easy for a scientific programme, especially a medical one, to go beyond the limits of education and touch the limits of alarm. This would have disastrous effects on a child's relationship with any sort of health care education, and fear of medicine often results from trauma during childhood.

Children are extremely sensitive and vulnerable and they are also able to understand much more than adults believe. This should be the starting point of every sort of education. To underestimate children's intelligence and understanding and to overestimate their resistance to harmful messages are common mistakes which ignore the uniqueness of a child's nature and personality.

RECOMMENDATIONS

In any consideration of the ability of very young children to observe, learn, and absorb attitudes and lifestyles, their tendency to mimic the many messages thrust upon them from family, school, community, and television, we must examine the practical steps which can be taken so that the influences operating early in life will lead them to adopt healthy lifestyles. And, equally important for the purpose of this book, we must decide how to proceed in this field without any infringment of generally accepted ethical values.

The first and most important recommendation from which everything else derives is to make everyone aware of the fact that *all children from infancy onwards can be influenced in a positive or negative way by everything that happens around them*. And since, as we said above, 'around them' are the members of the family, those working in day-care facilities, and the television screen, we discuss here the three environmental influences one by one.

First come *the parents* and others in the family. They have the responsibility and they have the authority, and no other individual or agency has the right to dictate or intervene, except obviously in suspected cases of abuse and neglect which are not relevant to our present discussion. The vital element here is education, and above all education that everything they do in the presence of their children, no matter how young they are, may have some influence on their present and future behaviour, including habits beneficial or detrimental to their health. It is quite common to hear a mother, when advised to avoid something in the presence of her young child, protest 'But he is too young to understand.' This is simply not true. Nobody can claim with any certainty that a child is too young, if not consciously to understand, at least unconsciously to absorb some message.

The way to reach and educate present and future parents will inevitably vary from country to country and will depend on the social and educational level of the family and on the facilities available. It will also depend on whether the curriculum of the schools the parents themselves attended did or did not contain instruction on child development, parental roles and responsibilities, and health education as such. Use should be made of schools for parents, where they exist, community groups, radio and television educational programmes, articles in the press, special journals for parents. They should also be advised that not only they, but all others in the family—grandparents, siblings, etc.—may play an equally important role, the more so if both parents are regularly away from home at work or elsewhere.

The personnel of day-care facilities have been trained for their task. Our attention should therefore be directed to the curriculum of their school. Does it contain lessons on health education? And above all does it sensitize the students to the fact that all their acts may be copied by the small children? Their behaviour in the nursery school, whether they realize it or not, whether they intend it or not, exerts some influence on the infants and young children under their care. In this respect a close cooperation between parents and preschool teachers is desirable, and various ways to achieve this have been described by Woodhead.[24]

Finally, we come to *television*. We have tried to explain earlier why the power of this new source of messages is so great. So what should be done about it? Inevitably advice and expertise in this area must come from individuals who are not only experts in mass communication media but also from professionals, acting individually or collectively, who are experts in the many aspects of child development, health education, and mental health.

REFERENCES

1. Spitz, R.A. Anaclitic depression. *The Psychoanalytic Study of the Child*. 1946; 2: 313–342.
2. Freud, A. *The Psycho-Analytical Treatment of Children*. London: Imago, 1946.
3. Bowlby, J. *Maternal Care and Mental Health*. Geneva: World Health Organization, 1951.
4. Holt, K.S. *Developmental Paediatrics*. London: Butterworths, 1977.
5. Doxiadis, S. (ed.). *Early Influences Shaping the Individual*. London: Plenum, 1989.
6. Schaffer, H.R. *The Child's Entry into a Social World*. London: Academic Press, 1984.
7. Hetzel, B.S. and Berenson, G.S. (eds.). *Cardiovascular Risk Factors in Childhood: Epidemiology and Prevention*. Amsterdam: Elsevier, 1987.
8. Huston, A.C., Wright, J.C., Kerkman, D., Seigle, J., Rice, N. and Bremen, M. Family Environment and Television Use by Preschool Children. Paper presented at the biennial convention of the Society for Research in Child Development, Detroit, 1983.
9. Anderson, D.R., Lorch, E.P., Erickson Field, D. and Sanders, J. The effects of TV program comprehensibility on preschool children's visual attention to television. *Child Dev* 1981; 52: 151–157.
10. Collins, W.A., Sobol, B.L. and Wesby, S. Effects of adult commentary on children's comprehension and inferences about a televised aggressive portrayal. *Child Dev* 1981; 52: 158–163.

11. Friedrich, L.K. and Stein, A.H. Prosocial television and young children: the effects of verbal labeling and role playing on learning and behavior. *Child Dev* 1975; **46**: 27–38.
12. US National Institute of Mental Health. *Television and Behavior. Ten Years of Scientific Progress and Implications for the Eighties*. Washington DC: Government Printing Office, 1982.
13. Postman, N. *The Disappearance of Childhood: How TV Is Changing Children's Lives*. London: Comet Books, 1985.
14. Natapoff, J.N. Children's views of health: a developmental study. *Am J Publ Health* 1987; **68**: 995–1000.
15. Feldman, F., Feldman, E. and Goodman, J.T. Culture versus biology: children's attitudes towards thinness and fatness. *Pediatrics* 1988; **81**: 190–194.
16. Goldstein, J. *Who Speaks for the Child*. New York, London: Plenum Press, 1982.
17. Council of Europe. *Parental Responsibilities*. Recommendation No. (84) 4, Principle 1, 1984.
18. Mill, J.S. *On Liberty*. Harmondsworth: Penguin Classics, 1985.
19. Freud, A., Goldstein, J. and Solnit, A. *Beyond the Best Interests of the Child*. New York: The Free Press, 1973.
20. Hewer v. Bryant. *3 All England Law Reports*, p. 578, 1969.
21. Feinbloom, R. Quoted in Culkin, J. (ed.) *Selling to Children: Fair Play in TV Commercials*. Hastings Center Report, 1978.
22. Culkin, J. (ed.). *Selling to Children: Fair Play in TV Commercials*. Hastings Center Report, 1978.
23. Karpf, A. *Doctoring the Media*. London: Routledge, 1988.
24. Woodhead, M. *Cooperation between Parents, Preschool and the Community*. Strasbourg: Council of Europe, 1987.

CHAPTER 9

Health Education in Schools

R. S. DOWNIE AND CAROL FYFE

SUMMARY

'Health' is a suitable subject for inclusion in a school curriculum. Moreover, to the extent that it satisfies certain criteria, and avoids certain ethical pitfalls, it can be seen as part of 'education properly so-called'. These criteria concern the knowledge base, the use of person-respecting methods, and the justification for health education. Typical ethical problems relate to the fact that health is an integral part of a total individual, familial, and communal lifestyle, and health education may create discord for a child within that lifestyle.

INTRODUCTION

In many ways the school is the ideal setting for education about health, but there are ethical and educational issues which ought to be considered. These issues arise less from the overall aim of health education—which is always to optimize health status—than from the specific objectives of health education in a school context. The objectives will vary according to the age and educational abilities of the pupils, and according to the educational contexts in which health education is pursued. For example, health education can refer to attempts to reinforce healthy behaviour patterns or improve health status, to the provision of simple information on health determinants and the availability of health services, and to more advanced study of health through basic biology and sociology. This diversity of legitimate objectives is further complicated by a new stress on the concept of positive health or well-being and on the development of self-esteem. The claim of health education to be a school subject with any or all of these objectives clearly raises educational and ethical problems of content, method, and justification. Our chapter will develop some of the points made in Recommendation No. R (88)7 by the Committee

Ethics in Health Education
Edited by S. Doxiadis. ©1990 John Wiley & Sons Ltd

of Ministers to Member States of the European Economic Community in their recent recommendation on School Health Education and the Role and Training of Teachers.

HEALTH EDUCATION AND PREVENTION

Before we raise our central questions, of whether health education is properly to be regarded as an appropriate subject for a school curriculum and of the possible ethical objections to it, we should perhaps deal with a preliminary objection. This objection will not easily strike those engaged in health education or health promotion because they are so familiar with the benefits of these activities. But it will occur to the majority of the general public who still think in terms of a medical model of health. Is health education really necessary? In school at least is the best policy not an effective programme of immunization and vaccination, supplemented perhaps with some frank warnings on the dangers of AIDS? Is anything more not just gratuitous preaching? The reply to this objection will enable us to begin our account of why health education is a necessary part of a school curriculum.

Within the area of primary prevention it is possible to distinguish activities aimed at protection against specific diseases and those aimed at providing more general protection. In the first category we can place the many activities and methods designed to prevent the occurrence or spread of specific diseases such as diphtheria, tetanus, poliomyelitis, and many other infectious diseases. Campaigns of this kind provide benefits to individuals (although in a small number of cases they have also harmed individuals) and to communities. The campaigns have a number of characteristics of which we shall mention four: (1) they are effective only with diseases which have a specific and known causation, (2) it must be possible to intercept the causation of the disease by using a specific immunization or vaccination, (3) the recipients of the vaccines do not need to understand what has been done to them but may be entirely passive, (4) the campaigns can be carried out cheaply and on a large scale. We might say that such campaigns have 'magic bullet' appeal which for many people expresses the scientific mystique of modern medicine.

The limitations of this approach to primary prevention are that most of the major health threats in present day society cannot be stopped by 'magic bullets', for the reason that they do not have the four characteristics of infectious diseases just mentioned.[1] The major health problems in the contemporary industrialized world are heart disease, stroke, cancer, accidental injuries (street and domestic), violence, child abuse, war. The causation in such cases is multifactorial and *may not be wholly known*. It follows from the nature of multifactorial causation that there cannot be any *specific* ways of intercepting it. Moreover, since the conditions may be behaviourally induced their prevention requires the *understanding* or at least the active cooperation of the individuals at risk to bring about changes in lifestyle.

But changes in lifestyle are not likely to be brought about *without a considerable cost* to the individual and society.

The activities, directed at encouraging this more general prevention of disease and ill-health through change in lifestyle, are at least part of what has come to be called 'health promotion', of which health education is one aspect.[2] Now if the major health problems of the contemporary world cannot be combated with 'magic bullets' but only by a 'lifestyle' approach, then the foundations of a healthy lifestyle should be encouraged as early as possible—in the school. This gives us our first argument for the inclusion of 'health' as a school topic; traditional prevention of a medical kind is not sufficient and health education in schools is a useful substitute.

HEALTH AND EDUCATION

To argue that 'health' should be a part of the school curriculum does not enable us to conclude that it is part of the child's *education*. Many activities take place in a school of a desirable nature which are not part of 'education', except in the trivial sense that they take place in an educational institution. For example, within the total activities of a school we might distinguish:

1. Education properly or narrowly so-called—mathematics, literature, science, history, and so on.
2. Subjects of mainly occupational relevance—typing, technical drawing, or computing.
3. Subjects concerned with social skills—dancing or dressmaking.
4. Moral and religious subjects.
5. The arts.
6. Sport and gymnastics.
7. Extracurricular activities—debating, climbing, and chess-playing.
8. Ancillary teaching or advising on careers, friendships, etc.
9. The necessary conditions of the above—in the primary school subjects of learning to read, write, and count.

Now these overlapping categories can no doubt be distinguished in various ways, and it would be very controversial in some contexts as to which activities are to be included as 'education properly so-called'. For example, in Britain an A-level or Scottish 'Higher' pass in Music is recognized as a subject which may count towards university entrance whereas an A-level pass in Art is not. Is Music part of 'education' but not Art? Fortunately, we need not, for our purposes, argue this point. We are insisting only on a less controversial point: that there are various types of activity going on in schools and not all of them are education properly so-called, although they may be very desirable in other respects, such as giving immediate enjoyment or having occupational relevance—more desirable, indeed, in these respects than some subjects which are part of 'education' proper. Our question is where 'health' fits in as a school subject. Can it be regarded as part of 'education properly so-called', or is it just a highly desirable part of the school curriculum?

It might be said of course that this question is of purely theoretical interest. The important point is that 'health' should be a part of the curriculum, and the question of whether or not it belongs to the class of subjects which are 'education properly so-called' is of secondary importance and can be left to philosophers of education. We do not accept this. If we can make a case for claiming that 'health' is part of education properly so-called we shall be making a contribution to enhancing the importance of 'health' in the eyes of pupils, their parents, their teachers, and those who fund education in schools. The question is therefore a theoretical one of great practical relevance. We shall accordingly devote most of the remainder of this chapter to the question of whether activities in school to encourage the development in children of a desirable attitude to health can be considered educational in a reasonably narrow sense. This will of course involve some attention to the ethical basis of such activities.

The question of what makes an activity 'educational' is complex and controversial, but the following factors are relevant to any discussion:

1. What is the quality of the knowledge base involved? If an activity is to be appropriately called 'educational' it must have some sort of accredited content, and the question is whether health education or health promotion does have that.
2. What are the methods used? Philosophers of education have often distinguished between 'education', 'instruction', 'training', and so on. Such distinctions are important for certain purposes, although we shall not insist on them here. Nevertheless, to be an 'educational' activity some sort of person-respecting methods must be used. The question is whether they are at present employed in health education and health promotion in school. A connected question concerns the position of the teacher. In education proper the teacher is not urging his own values but is neutrally presenting the evidence and arguments for various points of view. Does this happen in health education?
3. What sorts of justification can be offered for carrying out health education in schools? Are there ethical objections? Assuming that there are no fatal ethical objections to teaching 'health' in schools should it be done because 'health' is useful to the individual, or to the community? Or because being healthy is in some way worthwhile for its own sake? Is it just to cut down on community health bills? Or some combination of these?

Ethical questions come up especially over the questions of justification, but we shall not attempt to confine them to that part of our discussion. They will occur in all sections.

THE KNOWLEDGE BASE OF HEALTH EDUCATION

One of the difficulties involved in educating about health is that the knowledge base changes very rapidly and there are limited areas in which recommendations can be made on a factual basis.[3] Now it is true that knowledge changes in all subject areas. New words are persistently being introduced to all languages, changing the vocabularies being taught in schools. Similarly, in science subjects discoveries of new biological species, or new chemical elements, or new mathematical properties, must be incorporated into teaching materials. A changing knowledge base is therefore not a problem in principle for education. In practice, however, the problem is worse in the area of health than in other areas. Because health behaviours are entrenched in lifestyle, and health education involves value judgments, the incorporation of new information does not simply necessitate a change in people's knowledge about health, but also a change in lifestyle. While learners are reasonably open to accommodating new information, they are much more resistant to changing their lifestyle according to each new research discovery. Health educators are extremely aware of this and must be critical of research findings to establish their reliability before incorporating new messages into education.

While adults and adolescents may be able to assess new information, younger children are less able to be critical. In other words, simpler rather than complex messages must be employed—without teachers losing sight of the overall target of good education. Only a limited range of health messages may be accessible to children in the early stages of education, and health educators in schools may be obliged to overcome this problem by presenting an incomplete account of the state of knowledge about health.

For younger children in schools, then, health education will consist of simple messages and only limited information. Clearly, given these restrictions there may be only a limited number of health education topics and educational methods which can be applied to young children in schools.

Another restriction of content concerns views on the 'suitability' of some health-related topics for young children. It has been argued that education about cigarette smoking and illegal drugs, for example, has the effect of encouraging children to experiment with these substances. Therefore education about these topics should wait until the children are old enough to know better. Similarly, there is a belief that sex education merely encourages sexual promiscuity and should be delayed until the children are of an age at which the legal system permits sexual activity. By this time, however, it may be too late and children may already have distorted ideas.

The decision about the age at which children should receive education on various health topics should be made by referring to the extensive, and expanding, literature on the subject. Research into cigarette smoking behaviour among schoolchildren in the United Kingdom, for example, has shown that children start experimenting with cigarettes when they are about 10–11 years old.[4] Before this age only very small proportions have tried a cigarette. Therefore health education dealing with cigarette smoking is directed towards children of this age. Research has also shown, however, that patterns of smoking behaviour vary greatly between schools, and teachers are recommended to assess the picture within their particular school to determine the relevant stage of intevention.[5]

It is appropriate to mention here the trend that has taken place within health education away from the preventive topic-orientated approach to the more modern lifeskills approach.[6] The aim is to teach children how to cope with situations to enhance their general well-being. It incorporates political and societal dimensions, rather than being based on a purely medical model. Using this modern approach it is not so relevant to ascertain a complex picture of the pattern of health behaviours within each school, but it is crucial to arm children with lifeskills from an early age, in order that they can cope with situations whenever they arise.

Health education in schools needs to be flexible in content not only to deal with a wide range of ages of children, but also to accommodate the variety of health needs found within each age group. Inevitably education tends to be targeted at some hypothetical 'average' or 'normal' child, and this occurs within all educational subjects. Individual teachers are then responsible for tailoring their lessons to meet the range of needs and abilities within their class.

The problem is particularly acute for teachers educating about health. Firstly, the teachers may really be dealing with life-or-death topics depending on how their messages are received, understood, and acted upon. It is particularly important that health lessons are successful in making pupils truly value their health. As stated above, there is always the danger that the provision of information results in experimentation with dangerous substances. There is also the danger that health education is seen as an attempt to regulate and standardize lifestyles, and thus result in rebellious behaviour—the contrary effect to that at which we are aiming. This is a problem of accommodating the various personality types within a class and dealing with peer pressure.

There is a second problem related to the various health needs of children. We have argued that teachers should assess the needs within their own school and tailor their curriculum accordingly. In addition to assessing the behaviour patterns that are 'normal' for their school, teachers should also note the range of behaviours—especially the exceptions to the rule. It may not be acceptable to take a utilitarian viewpoint, in which we develop health education for the greatest good for the greatest number (although this is usually the criterion used by researchers evaluating the effectiveness of programmes). An alternative approach is to direct education at those who are *most at risk* of adopting anti-health behaviours. We can examine this approach by using education about cigarette smoking as an example. There is some evidence that the younger children start to smoke cigarettes, the more likely they are to be smokers in adult life.[7] Therefore the children who start smoking at the earliest age form an 'at risk' group. Health education would thus be targeted not at the age group when the majority of children start smoking but instead at children of the youngest age group at which we know children start to experiment with cigarettes.

Children not only exhibit a variety of health-related behaviours, they also have multiplicity of health status. A class of children is likely to contain some children with chronic illnesses, such as asthma and diabetes, as well as children with acute illness or injury. In addition to such specific, diagnosed illnesses, health status is known to be affected by social, economic, and housing circumstances. As we shall discuss in more detail later, health education should deal with these issues, illustrating environmental influences on health and discussing how healthful behaviour varies according to health status. Children suffering from chronic illness should see the health education as relevant to them rather than viewing themselves as exceptions to the rules.

Schools have a responsibility to provide health education that is relevant not only to the 'average' child in each age group but rather to *all* the children. Therefore, health education must be sufficiently flexible in content to accommodate the range of needs within each class. Teachers must also be aware of the sensitivity required in order that pupils exhibit healthful responses to their health messages rather than rebelling against them. But these qualifications do not disturb the basic claim that there is a solid knowledge base to health education and that therefore it satisfies the first condition for being included in the list of subjects which make up 'education properly so-called'.

There is, however, a further complexity in the question of the knowledge base of health education. The educational activities so far described in this section are mainly aimed at helping pupils to avoid ill-health rather than at the creation of health in a positive sense. A World Health Organization (WHO) document on health promotion states that its

'perspective is derived from a conception of "health" as the extent to which an individual or group is able, on the one hand, to realize aspirations and *satisfy* needs; on the other hand, to change or cope with the environment. Health is, therefore, seen as a resource for everyday life, not the objective of living; it is a positive concept emphasizing social and personal resources; as well as physical capacities.'[8]

If we grant that the aim of health education and health promotion should be thus positively conceived as the promotion of the wholeness of a person, his 'healing', or his well-being, what follows about the nature of the skills and expertise required to promote it? The obvious implication is that the skills and expertise will be so varied that no one team, far less an individual, will be able to possess them all. What is required is a cooperative or collective exercise. It will be a cooperative exercise, moreover, of considerable breadth. To bring this out, consider the connections between health and welfare and between negative and positive health.

First of all, health is clearly one very important part of welfare in that is is reasonably wanted for its own sake and in that possession of it is a necessary condition for pursuing very many other goals. The second connection between health and welfare is of course the dependence of mental and physical health on other aspects of welfare, both material and non-material. To take an obvious example, it is notorious that mental and physical health can be affected by enjoyment and well-being at school or college. There is a continuum here from children who develop colds or headaches through fear or dislike of a teacher or of a subject to students who break down or commit suicide through misery and feelings of inadequacy at college.

There is then an expertise involved in education about health negatively conceived, but health in this sense is just part of a wider concept of 'wholeness', well-being, or positive health. Various professions share in the expertise required to promote health in this full sense, and the entire enterprise can fairly be regarded as in a broad sense educational.

EDUCATIONALLY ACCEPTABLE METHODS

The second criterion which 'health' must satisfy to count as an educationally justifiable procedure is that it must employ person-respecting methods, encourage person-respecting behaviour, and indeed encourage self-respect or self-esteem. This is partly a matter of educational technique, of encouraging the growth of a critical faculty and learning actively by experience, but it is mainly an ethical matter, of treating learners as centres of rational consciousness with their own feelings and perspective on the world and not just as a set of reaction tendencies.

It might be thought to follow from this criterion that a teacher should be value-neutral on his subject matter. He should not seek to enforce his own point of view, but should rather act as a sort of chairman listening to differing arguments, or (as Socrates put it) he should act as a midwife, helping the birth process of his pupils 'ideas'. If that does follow then there is a difficulty, for teachers of health education cannot hold a neutral position. They must be committed to health as a value and regard certain health-related behaviours as good, others as bad. In health education, teachers cannot simply present facts relating to exercising, healthy eating, decision-making skills, and so on; they must also make clear that these activities *should be adopted* by their pupils, that they should become an established part of their lifestyle.

In this way health is different from other subject matters in the school curriculum. If we make a comparison with religious education, the difference is clear. Teachers of religious education will present facts and the history of various religions without believing that their pupils should adopt them, and although the teacher him or herself may be committed to one religion it is inappropriate to take a moral stand and state that one religion is *better* than others. Teachers of health education, on the other hand, must take a moral stance and explain why some behaviour patterns *are* better than others. There is no other subject on the curriculum which is so value-driven.

Some health educators have taken a different point of view. Let us take the example of what is called in health education literature 'values-clarification'. This term refers to processes by which a person or group can be assisted in finding out what their values really are. There are various methods which can be used to bring about a clarification of this kind, and some are mentioned by Ewles and Simnett.[9] For example, people might be encouraged to write down and rank activities they enjoy, or they might be asked to state the arguments in favour of something they enjoy, or they might be asked to state the arguments in favour of something they felt strongly about. Again, role-play or games may be used to encourage groups to become clear on their values. Now the details of these procedures are very important for practical purposes, and attention would need to be given to the way in which they might be deployed in schools, but we are more interested in the principles and assumptions behind them.

Ewles and Simnett[9] write as follows:

'Traditional teaching operates in the hope that the "right" attitudes and values will be "caught" by learners. In contrast, we suggest that health education requires people to think critically about their values and build up their own value system'. (p. 132)

Social work literature in a similar vein suggests that in dealing with clients it is important to be 'non-judgmental'. Now if the assumption here is that any set of values is as good as any other then it is not an assumption which is consistent with health education or health promotion, or indeed any sort of education whatsoever. Certainly, it is important that people should be encouraged to think critically about their values, and although our predecessors in health education did not have such imaginative methods as are nowadays recommended for values-clarification, there is no reason to think that the encouragement of critical appraisal has not always been part of health education. What does need to be questioned however is the phrase 'build up their own value system' and the correlative idea of the non-judgmental attitude.

Our view is that health education and health promotion are activities committed to a certain philosophy of the nature of the self and what makes it flourish, and to views of a well-ordered society. No doubt there are a large number of acceptable ways of living one's life, all of which will lead to the flourishing of human personality, but not every way is equally acceptable in health education. Similarly, there are no doubt several acceptable forms of social and political organization, but not every way is acceptable to those involved in health education. If these positions are not shared by health educators and health promoters, then why adopt slogans such as 'Be all you can be' or why stress the importance of books such as the *Black Report*[10] or *The Health Divide?*[11] In other words, health educators cannot consistently accept the 'sneer' quotes in Ewles and Simnett's phrase ' "right" attitudes', for health educators must believe that there are right attitudes to the individual and to society, or go out of business.

It is a totally different point what methods or procedures should be adopted to change attitudes in individuals or societies. Consider this analogy. A Christian missionary is not likely to be very successful if he arrives among a heathen tribe and declares 'All have sinned!' He may be committed to believing this, but he would be well-advised to live and work among the people and learn about their ways of life and their difficulties before he tries to change their attitudes. In a similar way, it may be counterproductive to preach too much about giving up smoking; but, all the same, a health educator is committed to the view that such a practice is objectively a bad practice. Again, there may be some doubt as to whether jogging is a desirable form of exercise in all, or indeed in any circumstances; but there can be no doubt that taking a moderate amount of regular exercise is objectively a good form of activity and should be part of a good life. In the area of political values there can be room for difference about the relative importance of values such as liberty and equality, but in health education we are surely committed to the view that the extent of the health divide between rich and poor in, say, contemporary Britain is wrong. But it is a *different* question, of political tactics, how this state of affairs is best changed.

To sum up this discussion of the neutral teacher, we are maintaining three principles: (1) that it is important to encourage pupils to clarify their own values about health and lifestyle, (2) that the methods used in doing this should be flexible and imaginative, (3) that teachers of health education are committed by their profession to the belief that there are right and wrong attitudes to life and its values, and in this last sense they are not neutral. But we see nothing in these principles which is contrary to the idea of education as a person-respecting process.

In this context it is appropriate to contrast two approaches to health education which can be presented as rivals. One stresses the importance of a cognitive core in the content, of rational argument and the provision of information on health determinants, with the aim of enabling people to make up their own minds. This approach has the autonomy of the individual as its supreme value and is much influenced by the important educational philosophy of R.S. Peters.[12] The obvious objection to an exclusive reliance on this approach is that is entirely unrealistic in a health context. People, especially young people, are not the rational choosers depicted. They are causally influenced by a host of factors in their upbringing, environment, and perhaps especially they are influenced by the images of young people created by wealthy companies with unhealthy products to sell. The other approach can be seen as a sort of behavioural extension of preventive medicine.[3] The aim here is to bring about behavioural change in children through affecting their beliefs and attitudes. But this approach, whether or not it is effective and whether or not it is more appropriate for adult audiences, does not sit easily within the context of education.

But the dilemma of an unrealistic rational approach or an uneducational causal approach is spurious; we are not faced with an either/or situation. Certainly, health education in schools, especially at the more senior level, involves 'values-clarification' on the part of the students, but equally the teacher must be prepared to make her commitment to certain values apparent, and must be prepared to try to make these values as attractive as possible. Health educators ought not to be involved in a policy of 'must not do', but ought to try, perhaps via young persons' role models, to influence their health behaviour. Why should the devil have all the good tunes? A middle course will enable health education to influence behaviour but also keep it within the sphere of acceptable educational method.

Recent work in developing the health education curriculum in the United Kingdom has taken an intermediate approach of this type, based on broad educational principles. The Schools Council Health Education Projects 5–13 and 13–18 for primary and secondary schools form a notable example.[13] These projects are based on the belief that health education is largely concerned with influencing behaviour. Affecting health knowledge by the provision of information is not enough (although this traditional role of health education must not be abandoned).[14] Health behaviour is seen to derive from the processes of socialization and, therefore, in order that health education will affect behaviour it, too, must make a positive contribution to socialization.

The approaches taken in these Schools Council Projects go beyond the purely 'educational', as narrowly defined. They acknowledge that young people, because of peer-group pressures, false consciousness, lack of opportunities, and other factors, cannot always exercise free rational choice. The emphasis is therefore on the self-government of individuals through the teaching of lifeskills which develop self-esteem or self-respect and on decision-making skills. Young people with such skills are better able to resist pressures to conform, and to be more aware of their value in the community. In other words, free, rational choice becomes an objective rather than an assumption.

The Schools Council Projects were developed to cover the range of ages throughout primary and secondary schools, and emphasis was placed on providing appropriate inputs (in terms of the nature of content) at appropriate times. Projects of this type require extensive coordination between schools and among teachers within schools.

Other projects have also adopted a lifeskills approach but have been developed for one particular age group of children. For example, the Health Education Council's *My Body* project[15] and the *Jimmy on the Road to Superhealth* project,[16] funded by the Cancer Research Campaign, were developed for children aged 10–12, in upper-primary-school classes. These projects have been found to effect significant changes in behaviour.[17,18] Epidemiological evidence of this type provides welcome support for our theoretical advocacy of a broader approach to health education in schools.

Having stated and interpreted our views on the neutrality of health education, however, we must also admit that some of the practice of health education requires defence against the charge that it does not use person-respecting methods. Sometimes this defence is successful and sometimes it remains weak. Take, for example, the charge that health education in schools sometimes involves political indoctrination and in this respect is therefore not person-respecting. Now it is true that some health education approaches take an overtly political stance. Examples include discussions of governments' roles in promoting unhealthy products through advertising, and because of the taxation benefits. Publications such as *The Smoke Ring*[19] identify the roles of specific named members of parliament in endorsing unhealthy products. Does discussion of the political dimensions of health involve indoctrination?

Different models and conceptions of health have resulted in a range of alternative views about the remit of health education. It is, therefore, important for health educators to clarify the parameters of their concerns if they are to be effective in practice. Now, it is widely known that the influences on health are multifactorial, and include environmental and political factors. Indeed it has been stated that the *fundamental* determinants of health and health care are political.[20] If we accept the importance of political influences on health, we should then accept that discussion of these influences should play a role in health education.

It does not follow, however, that the inclusion of a political aspect turns health education into indoctrination. Person-respecting methods must still be used, and the distinction between 'politics' and 'party-politics' remembered. Education about the political aspects of health must involve the learners in critical assessment of the facts, not merely unquestioning acceptance of one particular viewpoint. Young people are certainly able to understand and assimilate arguments concerning the role of advertising, the political sway of large multinational companies, and so on. Discussions about these issues should certainly be a component of health education in schools, and cannot reasonably be thought to offend against the ethical requirements of educational method. Obviously such discussions are suitable only for more advanced pupils.

Contrary to the fear of the inclusion of political dimensions within health education is the argument that health education in schools at present does not take a *sufficiently* political stance. Cribb[21] describes the forces which press towards a conservative curriculum. These include the examination system, the lobby for traditional academic subjects, the argument that education should be relevant to the marketplace, and the stress placed on the primacy of basic expository skills. He argues, however, that schools are not independent from politics, that teachers should examine and become self-conscious about the values which they are transmitting to their pupils, that 'teaching for political literacy is not only different from the transmission of ideologies, it is a positive safeguard against it' (p. 114).

We would agree with this view. Young people are being exposed to many influences which are not free from bias and distortion, and a role of school health education should be to raise their critical awareness of these issues. It should not merely sweep them under the carpet.

Children being educated to value health must consider all aspects and the range of known determinants of health. Health education should change their way of looking at things which influence health, and thus must include a political stance. We have stated above that health educators must be committed to health as a value, they cannot hold a neutral stance. Similarly, they must be prepared to become involved in the political arena where this influences health. A political stance within health education is not encouraging an anti-establishment youth but, rather, a youth culture which is aware of health as general well-being and of influences on health beyond the purely medical.

JUSTIFICATIONS: VALUING HEALTH

Our discussion under this heading will be in two overlapping parts: one part will be negative, defending health education in schools against two objections to its inclusion in the curriculum, and the other will be positive, bringing out the positive reasons in its favour.

The first objection to health education in schools concerns the possible conflict which it can create in the home.[22] Because health is deeply entrenched in lifestyle the child will inevitably be exposed to the health behaviours of significant others in the home. These may conflict with the values passed on to him at school, with those health behaviours which he has been educated to believe are the better ways to follow. There are several possible consequences of this to be considered.

Firstly, rather than the school health education being reinforced out of school it will be diluted or negated by contradictory experience in the home. Therefore many of the teacher's efforts may be wasted, and the effectiveness of school health education greatly reduced. But this situation is little different from that in many subjects where the home reality is discordant with the messages taught in school. The discrepancy between the 'Queens English' taught in schools and the colloquialisms and dialects prevalent in society is a clear example of this. In other words, this constitutes a problem, but not one peculiar to health education in schools.

Secondly, when faced with behaviours in the home which are discordant with those they have been taught to value, children may undertake to educate their family about health and thereby pass on the values they have learnt in school. This could possibly cause conflict in the home. Family members might view the child as taking the establishment viewpoint and turning against the family and their daily experience. The child then is open to exclusion and rejection in the home. On the other hand, a child undertaking to educate his or her family about health could have some positive outcomes. The effects of school health education can go far beyond the school walls. It is useful here to distinguish between family health education undertaken at the child's own initiative, and that aimed at by health educators in schools. The situation we have postulated above arises from the child him or herself choosing to attempt to effect change in the behaviours of family members. Clearly these attempts may be successful or could cause family conflict.

The second situation involves use of children by health educators to reach other family members.

Some health education packages for schools are specifically designed to use the child as a means of reaching and affecting the health behaviours of parents.[23] Intended outcomes include health education of the parents and reinforcement of the health education directed at the children. We have some reservations about this approach however. From the health educators' viewpoint it is an easy way to reach an otherwise relatively inaccessible adult population. While we wholeheartedly support the adoption of many approaches to health education, we would not endorse the use of children to compensate for health educators' difficulties in reaching sections of the adult population. Children then become pawns in a game of education in which the goal is to effect behaviour change among parents.

These approaches cannot accommodate the variety of home backgrounds in which children are brought up, nor can they have the sensitivity of the child's own awareness of the personalities and reactions of his or her family members. It seems much preferable to develop methods of school health education which are effective in making children value health sufficiently to be motivated to pass their values on to family members as and when they feel it is appropriate. In this way, children are not merely compliant participants within family health education but are using their own initiative and personal experience.

A second objection to health education is that it elevates health into an important value and this (it is claimed) will make for egocentricity. It might be compared to the spiritual self-absorption characteristic of some religious fanatics in earlier ages. In replying to this objection we must concede that an undue concern with physical health is a characteristic to be found in some present day societies, perhaps especially on the west coast of the United States. But to see health as a positive good is not necessarily to commit oneself to self-absorption. It is certainly the view of the WHO that positive health is 'seen as a resource for everyday life, not the objective of living'. This raises the question of the sense or senses in which health might be said to be a value, and in answering this question we shall pass to the second and more positive stage in our justification of health education in schools.

The answer to the questions why and in what senses health, physical and mental, is a value is quite complex. One reason why health is valuable is of course obvious; freedom from incapacitating physical or mental illness is valuable because it is useful; it enables the person who has that freedom to carry out his purposes, whatever these may be, and the same is true of freedom from incapacitating injury or deformity. There is no-one who does not have reason to want health for the usefulness of it, whatever his projects in life. It is generally regarded as important to learn how to read, write, and to do basic arithmetic. These are basic abilities which are necessary in order to cope with many situations and so it is worthwhile learning them. It is also generally regarded as important to maintain a certain level of health, for illness and disease often restrict ability to participate in society, to carry out a job of work, and so on. Therefore it is worthwhile to learn how to look after yourself. One widely recognized function of school education is just that.

But what we have said so far makes health valuable only as a means, not as an end, and so not a value in the positive sense with which we are now concerned. The second reason for valuing health, however, makes health valuable not for what it brings but for what it is: health is desirable because sickness is painful. We can amplify this point by recalling the positive pleasures—glows of fitness and so on—which attend the peak of health. This sort of justification of health education seems again to enable it to fall within the remit of a desirable school activity. The rewards of health in this sense may be subjective or objective: they may involve 'feeling better' within oneself or 'appearing better' to others. Of course the two are not mutually exclusive. Someone who has just won the pools may not only feel happy and excited themselves, they may also appear to be a better prospect to suitors, clients, or friends. Similarly, people spending time looking after their health often feel better within themselves, both physically and mentally, and may indeed have the additional aesthetic reward of 'a healthy glow'. If health education helps pupils to feel good about themselves, to have confidence in their bodies, then it can be justified. The concept of self-esteem is relevant here. It has been plausibly argued that if the pupils can be encouraged to feel that they matter and have a contribution to make they are more likely to develop a sense of responsibility. 'Feeling good' about oneself is a component of self-esteem.

It should be noted that if health is valued in this second way it is not being regarded as something to be approved of, but simply as something wanted for its own sake; it is being seen as a liking value rather than as an ideal value.[24]

It is also possible to value health in a third way; to regard it as an ideal to be sought after, in such a way that people who cherish health are to be approved of and people who squander it are to be disapproved of. Aristotle distinguished three types of thing which people desire: the useful, the pleasant, and the noble. Health can be desired under all three headings. It is easy to explain, as we have seen, how it can be desired under the first two. To explain the third is more difficult. But it is perhaps a biological and teleological or purposive idea of how our species is 'meant' to be which catches people's imaginations. It is partly also an aesthetic idea, of a design with which we ought to conform, and in terms of which aberrations are seen as ugly. People can dislike conditions in themselves, and see them as ugly, simply because they see them as unhealthy.

There are various ways of explaining this idea of health as an ideal. A secular approach might be in terms of respect for the species: it might be said that it is incumbent on us as human beings to make our human nature flourish. This is an idea which goes back to Plato, and it has perennial appeal. J.S. Mill[25] states it as follows:

'Human nature is not a machine to be built after a model, and set to do exactly the work prescribed for it, but a tree, which requires to grow and develop on all sides according to the tendency of the inward forces which make it a living thing.'

It is true that Plato and Mill were apt to see human nature in mainly intellectual terms. But one might with equal plausibility see a person as a mind/body unity; and even if it is in virtue of his intellect that Man is thought of as a superior species, this assessment once arrived at might seem to entail some reverence for the species of body which contains this intellect. At all events it is plausible to suggest that the value people place upon health *as such*, apart from both its usefulness and its pleasantness, makes it a kind of ideal value, creating strong feelings in some people. Plato was appealing to some such feeling when he said that justice could be shown to be valuable in itself, not only for its results, if it was seen as a *healthy* state of soul.

If health education in schools can inspire pupils with idealism of this sort then it is expressing the central tradition of western education. The critics of health education are quite wrong if they depict it as a new-fangled idea. The truth is rather that it belongs to the tradition of education founded on Plato's *Republic*. It is a Platonic ideal that education is of the whole man, and to include health education as a compulsory part of the curriculum is to ensure that education will be of the whole man.

JUSTIFICATIONS: INDIVIDUAL AND SOCIAL

Our justification for health education has so far concentrated on the good it will bring about for individual children. Is there any social good likely to come about through health education in school? There are obvious traditional justifications to be found for the exercise of health education by the state or state-funded bodies. It is a basic function of a government to protect its citizens from disease. There is no problem about this if we are thinking of infectious or contagious diseases. The most topical example of this is of course the vast nationwide campaign in the United Kingdom against AIDS. A great deal is known about how to avoid HIV infection and there is obvious justification for communicating this information to as wide a section of the community as possible. This is true even on the most minimalist views of the function of government, where the idea of 'harm to others' is the dominant one. There is therefore a social justification for health education in schools.

Relevant here is an aspect of the *methods* of health promotion which we did not touch on directly in the previous section. Legislation can be counterproductive and education is sometimes more effective. And one could add here that even were it the case that legislation might sometimes be effective there is still the question as to whether there can be too high a price to pay for the enforcement of principles which might in themselves be desirable. The general point is that liberalism is not simply about what ought or ought not to be enforced but also about ways of proceeding to convince people by education and example as to how they ought to behave towards others. The activities of health education can be effective here in persuading children to change their lifestyles, or in creating a social attitude which will be sympathetic to actual legislation. For example, the seat-belt compaign in the United Kingdom prepared the way for subsequent legislation, which is widely accepted.

The problem of finding a social justification for health education in schools becomes more acute when we turn from health negatively conceived to well-being or health positively conceived. Do schools, and indirectly the state, have any social as opposed to individual justification for using school time to promote or encourage by education positive health or well-being? One answer might be that if there is social justification for education directed at improving negative health there is also social justification for education directed at improving positive health. The claim is that the encouragment of positive health will bring about physical and mental states which are resistant or more resistant to disease agents. A claim of this sort needs a great deal of empirical evidence to support it, and in any case is always in danger of being made true by definition—if you succumb to ill-health then you did not have enough positive health. Nevertheless, at a common sense level it seems obviously true that if you are in general terms fit then you are less likely to succumb to disease, and if you do succumb to disease then you will recover more quickly if usually you enjoy 'positive health'. If therefore there is justification for the promotion of health in the negative sense the same justification holds for the promotion of positive health.

There is the possibility of another sort of social justification for including health education as a compulsory part of the school curriculum. This sort of justification applies equally to health negatively and positively conceived, and it highlights an aspect of health education which is undoubtedly part of 'education properly so-called'. This aspect concerns the social determinants of health.

It is now well-known that there are good correlations between health states and social class in all countries, although especially in Britain. What this means is that there is a significant health divide among members of one society. The idea of citizens with equal rights and responsibilities does not fit easily into societies so divided. It is now recognized by adherents of the political left and right alike (although for different reasons) that the cure for this division is not 'top-down' welfarist intervention and handouts but a 'bottom-up' growth of a sense of community. Health education can help here by encouraging discussion of the role of the community and self-help groups in spreading the idea of health for all. Certainly, the preamble to the Constitution of the WHO of 1946 asserts that there is a *right* to positive health. In ambitious terms it states, 'The enjoyment of the highest attainable standard of health is one of the fundamental rights of every human being without distinction of race, religion, political belief, economic or social condition.' If this is a fundamental right then presumably there is a correlative duty laid upon governments to implement it, and one way of doing this is to encourage education about health and its social determinants.

We shall conclude by putting our point in terms of grammar, as a change from the more usual sociological or medical models of health and health education.

Health can be and was traditionally seen as an *adjective*—a kind of attribute or property which individuals could possess, which could be protected by vaccination and impaired by disease. According to more recent ways of looking at health, health is an *adverb*—a style of living, a way of qualifying the active verbs of living. This is part of the promotional or lifestyle approach to health. But we want to suggest that health can also be seen as a *relational predicate*—that health and well-being can be seen as a set of relationships in which the community as a whole participate to obtain mutual benefits, benefits which include a decline in the rates of disease, fair access to health care, and some shared beliefs about a good life.[26]

It might be said that to think of health as an adverb, a lifestyle, or a relational predicate, a way of living with respect to others in a community, is to speak of health determinants rather than health itself; a certain style of life conduces to health, and a good community spirit conduces to health. But this objection begs the question—which is whether health is wholly reducible to the efficient biological functioning of an individual. Our view is that it is not reducible to individual concepts; it is not a metaphor to speak of health as expressible in social relationships.

Health education in schools can be immensely helpful here in spelling this out and bringing out in vivid ways to pupils their rights and responsibilities as citizens. These may be ideas remote from medical practice, and they may be seen as disturbingly revolutionary to some educationists or politicians, but in fact they are as old as Plato's *Republic*, and to base health education on ideas from that venerable book certainly places it within the sphere of 'education properly so-called'. Moreover, they are ideas which in general outline have been adopted as recently as 18 April 1988, by the Committee of Member States of the Council of Europe.[27]

CONCLUSION

Let us sum up this complex justification for including health education as a part of the school curriculum. We argued that not only was 'health' a suitable subject for inclusion in the school curriculum but that it could be seen as part of 'education properly or narrowly so-called'. First, it has a respectable, although developing, knowledge base which can be adapted to pupils of all ages. Secondly, it can employ person-respecting methods, although that does not mean either that it is value-neutral or that it is prohibited from using the wide range of techniques which teachers of all subjects employ to make their messages attractive to pupils. Thirdly, the teaching of 'health' can be justified on both an individual and a community basis. Health is useful to the individual, a necessary condition of much else; it is pleasant to its possessor, and in making its possessor 'feel good' it contributes to self-esteem and a sense of responsibility. From a social point of view health education can assist legislation, and more importantly it can lead to the development of a sense of community. Above all, health can be shown as an ideal value in its own right, as something to be approved of and defended. Just as 'quality of architecture' or 'a good natural environment' are expressions of values, so health in the individual and in the community as a whole is a value which is at the basis of Western civilization and Western education.

REFERENCES

1. Eisenberg, L. Social policies for promoting health. In Doxiadis, S. (ed.). *Ethical Dilemmas in Health Promotion*. Chichester: Wiley, 1987.
2. Tannahill, A. What is health promotion? *Hlth Educ J* 1985; **44**: 167–168.
3. Tones, B.K. Training needs for health education. *J Inst Hlth Educ* 1977; **15**: 22–29.
4. Goddard, E. and Ikin, C. *Smoking Among Secondary Schoolchildren in 1986*. London: OPCS, HMSO, 1987.
5. Charlton, A., Gillies, P. and Ledwith, F. Variations between Schools and Regions in Smoking Prevalence among British Schoolchildren—Implications for Health Education. *Publ Hlth* 1985; **99**: 243–249.
6. Tannahill, A. and Robertson, G. Health Education in Medical Education: Collaboration, not Competition. *Med Teach* 1986; **8**: 165–170.
7. McKennell, C.A. and Thomas, R.K. *Adults and Adolescents Smoking Behaviour and Attitudes*. Government Social Survey SS 353/13. London: HMSO, 1967.
8. WHO. *Health Promotion—A Discussion Document on the Concept and Principles*. Supplement to Europe News, No. 3. Copenhagen: WHO Regional Office for Europe, 1984.
9. Ewles, L. and Simnett, I. *Promoting Health. A Practical Guide to Health Education*. Chichester: Wiley, 1985.
10. Townsend, P. and Davidson, N. (eds) *Inequalities in Health: The Black Report*. Harmondsworth: Penguin, 1982.
11. Whitehead, M. *The Health Divide: Inequalities in Health in the 1980s*. London: Health Education Council, 1987.
12. Peters, R.S. *The Philosophy of Education*. Oxford: Oxford University Press, 1973.
13. Schools Council. *All About Me 5–8*. London: Nelson, 1977. *Think Well 9–13*. London: Nelson, 1977. *Health Education 13–18*. London: Forbes, 1982.
14. Reid, D. Into the mainstream. In Lee, J. (ed.) *A Guide to School Health Education*. London: Health Education Council, 1982.
15. Health Education Council and Sheffield L.E.A. *My Body Project Materials*. London: Heineman, 1983.
16. Calman, A.L.H., Carmichael, S., Deans, H.G. and Calman, K.C. Development of a primary school health education programme with special emphasis on the prevention of cigarette smoking. *Hlth Educ J* 1985; **44**: 65–69.
17. Gillies, P.A. and Wilcox, B. Reducing the Risk of Smoking Amongst the Young. *Publ Hlth Lond* 1984; **98**: 49–54.
18. Deans, G., Calman, A. and Carmichael, S. Smoking interventions in the primary school—some implications of an evaluation of a recently developed programme. Paper presented at the 2nd National Conference on Health Education and Youth, 6–12 September, University of Southampton, 1984.
19. Taylor, P. *The Smoke Ring: Tobacco, Money and Multinational Policies*. London: Sphere, 1985.
20. Scott-Samuel, A. The Politics of Health. *Comm Med* 1979; **1**: 123–126.
21. Cribb, A. Politics and health in the school curriculum. In Rodmell, S. and Watt, A.

(eds). *The Politics of Health Education—Raising the Issues*. London: Routledge and Kegan Paul, 1986.

22. Tones, B.K. Socialisation, health career and the health education of the schoolchild. *J Inst Hlth Educ* 1979; **17**: 23–28.

23. Charlton, A. evaluation of a family-linked smoking programme in primary schools. *Hlth Educ J* 1986; **45**: 140–144.

24. Downie, R.S. and Telfer, E. *Caring and Curing*. London: Methuen, 1980.

25. Mill, J.S. On liberty. In Warnock, M. (ed.). *Utilitarianism*. London: Collins, 1962.

26. Beauchamp, D. Lifestyle, public health and paternalism. In Doxiadis, S. (ed.). *Ethical Dilemmas in Health Promotion*. Chichester: Wiley, 1987.

27. Council of Europe Committee of Ministers. Recommendation No. R (88)7, *School Health Education and the Role of Training of Teachers*, 1988.

CHAPTER 10

Health Education and Self-Care

YANNIS C. TOUNTAS

SUMMARY

Health education, when aiming at the promotion of self-care, confronts a number of ethical issues. The first of these is that of the effectiveness of self-care, and more specifically of the effectiveness of health education in self-care, in order to be able to justify any support for self-care and more particularly for the implementation of health education programmes. The second issue is that of the distribution of limited resources and of the ethical issues that any relocation policy implies. The next issue involves the more general ideological and political implications of self-care and health education, and the last issue focuses upon the tension between autonomy and paternalism. In this chapter I will attempt to provide answers to some of the problems that arise in this area of health education and to describe the fundamental aspects of others.

INTRODUCTION

Self-care is one of the fundamental components in primary health care. As a sector which produces services in health promotion and in prevention as well as disease detection and treatment, it is involved in all the ethical issues which are related to those services. The significant difference which exists and which gives an even greater dimension to the moral aspect is that lay people, rather than health professionals, are responsible for providing the services.

An extensive ethical literature has developed around health education and its three basic activities: information provision, attitude and behaviour change, and environmental improvement. All the ethical issues related either to self-care or to health education have been recorded in detail in the many published studies. To list them would not only go beyond the scope of this chapter; it would also offer

Ethics in Health Education
Edited by S. Doxiadis. ©1990 John Wiley & Sons Ltd

us nothing new. However, there is a considerable need for our thinking to focus on the particular ethical issues which arise from the development of health education programmes in the field of self-care.

These particular ethical issues involve four central questions. The first of these is that of the effectiveness of self-care, and more specifically of the effectiveness of health education in self-care. Both of these sectors are concerned primarily with probable outcomes whose precise effects are often difficult to predict. This makes the choices much harder to assess from a moral viewpoint. However, we should deal first with the question of effectiveness, so as to be able to justify any support for self-care and more particularly for the implementation of health education programmes.

The second question is that of the distribution of existing resources. At a time when resources for health are limited, any relocation policy is an option with considerable moral implications.

The next question involves the more general ideological and political implications of self-care and the ethical issues which arise when health education, with the form and content of its programmes, cannot remain indifferent to these ideological and political implications.

The last question is a particularly important one; it focuses upon the tension between autonomy and paternalism. The self-care philosophy relies on autonomy and independence from iatrocentric thinking. How far is this autonomy brought about by the intervention of the health education services which have been institutionalized, and who decides about the needs, content, and techniques of a health education programme? The state? The health services? Community and societal agencies? Or the persons immediately concerned—that is, the self-care practitioners?

I shall try to provide specific thoughts and proposals on all these questions within the framework of this chapter. First of all, however, I would like to define the central concept—self-care.

SELF-CARE

Self-care could be defined as 'a process whereby a layperson functions on his/her own behalf in health promotion and prevention and in disease detection and treatment.'[1] It is neither a new nor a fringe phenomenon; it has been a fundamental aspect of health behaviour in human societies since their inception. Despite that, it is only in the last 15 or 20 years that self-care has stimulated extensive scientific attention. During that period, it has become clear that individuals are not just consumers of health services; they also pursue health and provide health care themselves through a broad range of activities. Also during this period a growing awareness of the societal production of illness and of the ineffectiveness of therapeutic medicine has led to a search for new or alternative approaches.

Within the framework of this thinking, self-care is seen today as the first level and the most pervasive form of primary health care.[2] All the other levels of professional health care supply are auxiliary and supportive. In reality, they are supplements to the health care provided by the individual or the family, which meets between 65% and 85% of the total requirements.[3,4]

However, over and above the individual and the family there are also various unions of individuals whose aim is that their members should mutually meet their own health needs. These unions, which we encounter relatively frequently today in the developed societies, can be in the form either of 'volunteer health care organizations' or of 'self-help groups.'[5] A simple definition of self-help might be 'groups of people who feel that they have a common problem and have joined together to do something about it.'[6] Such groups have small numbers of members and may involve themselves in dealing with a health problem, a disease, or a handicap.[7]

In all its manifestations, self-care may occupy at least three different positions in relation to the professional health system–it may function within the system, it may work in parallel to it, or it may operate in complete opposition to it.[5]

The specific sectors in which self-care has been applied and developed most extensively are those involving health problems such as obesity and alcoholism, chronic illnesses such as diabetes and asthma, mental disturbances such as schizophrenia and retardation, the rehabilitation of heart-attack sufferers and other chronic cases, and the encouragement of the handicapped and disabled to join the social, labour, and family environment.

However, no understanding of the self-care phenomenon will be complete if it confines itself to the framework of its specific applications. Apart from the realignments which it has brought about in the professional care system, self-care has had an effect on the more general evolution of social and natural systems of caring. In effect, what has occurred is a search for a new ecology of caring in society, one which is founded on the principles of self-reliance and self-determination.[5] These principles give individuals the potential to become aware of the health problems they have, to be able to manage them and subsequently to construct a new functional relationship of reconciliation with the specific problem. From that point of view, self-care is another way of life.

EFFECTIVENESS

The answer to the question 'what evidence exists to suggest any tangible benefits for individuals who subscribe to the self-care philosophy in order to justify the implementation of health education programmes?' is incomplete because of the scanty amount of research work which has been done on this topic. Measurement and assessment of health education programmes in the field of self-care have been even rarer.

Most research into the topic has observed positive results. The rehabilitation of heart-attack patients was considerably improved by their membership of self-help groups, with the participation of a health practitioner in the role of group leader.[8] A large-scale research project in Norway concluded that self-help groups made a particularly significant contribution to combating obesity in a population which had proved completely resistant to organized intervention on the part of the medical world.[9]

There were also considerable benefits from the implementation of health education programmes based on the team approach to self-help groups of diabetics,[10] to self-care programmes for dental and mouth care in children,[11] to care of the elderly,[12] and for instruction in breast self-examination among women of lower socioeconomic classes.[13]

On the other hand, some researchers in the field of mental health believe that self-care can produce positive results without a need for a theoretical knowledge of mental disturbance or the specialized therapeutic techniques that a health education programme could provide.[14]

Apart, however, from the measurement of effectiveness some other criteria have been proposed for the assessment of self-care. These include self-efficacy, sharing information with the client, client satisfaction, and active client involvement. Quite a number of studies, particularly those relating to the management of asthma in children, have concluded that these criteria were satisfactorily complied with in a range of self-care educational programmes.[1] Other related studies have shown a clear superiority for the contribution made by health education and self-care in cases of asthma among children by comparison with traditional forms of medical treatment.[15]

There have, of course, been self-care programmes which, when assessed, are seen to have produced no particular results, particularly in the area of therapy. Yet even in these cases, if we ignore the traditional medical criteria it will be seen that self-care has made a contribution by improving self-confidence, by the patient's loss of a sense of stigma, by combating loneliness, by managing day-to-day problems, and so on.

As a conclusion, it could be argued that self-care and the implementation of related health education programmes bring about a modest increase in public competence in health which has the clear potential for a powerful improvement in health indicators. In addition, by increasing competence in primary health care, we can arrive at the most effective, safest, most available, most acceptable and most economical way of meeting health needs.[16,17] We shall also have a potential reduction in the iatrogenic effects of professional care, particularly dependency. The social control of the medical care system is also reduced, liberating the humanitarian potential of the community and allowing the family, the church, and other agencies to contribute to the care and treatment of the public.

For all these reasons, support for self-care and its associated health care programmes should not be impeded or suspended for moral reasons connected with questioning of its effectiveness.

RESOURCE ALLOCATION

As soon as we have even partial evidence of the contribution made by self-care and its associated health education programmes, we have resolved, to some extent, the ethical issues which are connected with the policy of allocating the limited resources set aside for health. However, there are other aspects of this question which should not be allowed to pass without comment.

First of all, since in most cases there is no actual government policy towards self-care, when cuts in expenditure are being implemented it may appear questionable to pay more attention to voluntary work. Furthermore, the emphasis laid on the role of the individual might imply that citizens are about to be deprived of something without getting anything back in exchange.

If this is not the case and if there is a real will to help self-care, the first ethical issue which arises is that of the specific orientation of the support. Should it be a question simply of maximizing the anticipated health improvements, or ought such improvements to be distributed in ways that, for example, favour the most disadvantaged?

Another ethical problem related to the issues of distribution and equity arises from the fact that the participants in most self-care instruction programmes were, as one would expect, the most highly educated and articulate self-care practitioners. As a result, they captured a disproportionate share of professional attention and resources, perhaps even at the expense of less articulate people whose conditions might be more severe. This risk, if it does exist, is perhaps the exception rather than the rule, since for the most part self-care is an additional resource for health.

That, however, does not dispose of the ethical issue of equity raised by the claim that self-care should be supported out of the public purse. Nor, of course, is the issue answered by asserting that since self-care is voluntary anyone who wants can take part in it, because this is not the case. In the end, what has to be said is that making a place for self-care does not require material resources in excess of a tiny fragment of the total health budget and of the money spent on the development of high-technology medicine.

The resources requirements fall even further if we remember the numerous positive financial effects which the practice of self-care has, as shown by research in the area. Self-care education in the elderly is associated with a decrease in the use of medical facilities, with relative cost reduction.[18] A self-help programme run by the University of Southern California medical centre reduced by two-thirds the number of patients experiencing diabetic coma and saved hospitals and patients $1.4 million over a period of two years. A self-care programme for haemophiliacs at Tufts New England medical centre reduced the cost per patient by 45%.[19] In an educational programme for self-management skills among asthmatic children and their parents in an ambulatory care setting, estimated hospital and emergency room costs were significantly reduced.[20] On the other hand, a study of the impact of self-care education on health maintenance organization (HMO) costs did not demonstrate that the programme had any significant effect on the frequency or the total cost of clinic visits.[21]

In view of all the above, if the self-care movement is to work alongside professional providers of medical care then it must be seen more as an additional resource and less as an additional burden. From that point of view, the ethical issues should strengthen, not suspend, the support and development of self-care and the educational programmes with which it is associated.

IDEOLOGY AND POLITICS

The philosophy of self-care is not confined to concepts of meeting health requirements. It also extends to more general views about health, the ideology and politics of health systems, the emancipation of the individual, and some other issues which frequently bring self-care into ideological and political conflict with iatrocentric systems and with official medical science.

In the context of this conflict, the intervention of health education creates a series of ethical issues, given that it is called upon, directly or indirectly, to take up a position in favour of one or other approach. In this way, it is called upon first of all to declare its views on the question of the democracy and decentralization of the state. According to the Yugoslavian experience,

'self-care means decentralizing the loci of decision-making and state power in such a way as to ensure the aggregation and mutual adjustment of diverse social interests and resources *down* at the most basic units of social life; and the reverse to ensure an equal, democratic representation of pluralistic interests *upwards* in the system of sociopolitical management, from these basic social units all the way up to the state representation.'[22]

In the Soviet Union, voluntary social work is cherished by constitutional theory. The withering away of the state will be achieved, it is thought, only if people take an active part in government, the economy, health, and social welfare. Following these guidelines, self-care in the Soviet Union has grown significantly—to such an extent, indeed, that in many cases lay workers outnumber paid officials.[23]

In the socialist countries the philosophy of self-care may display a considerable number of points of correspondence with the dominant political ideology, but this is not the case in the capitalist states. In these latter countries the coexistence of a welfare state and of private enterprise in the health sector usually makes ordinary citizens passive consumers of the products and services turned out by the private or public sector.

It follows that one of the ethical questions which arises concerns the role of health education programmes: should they involve themselves with the strengthening or weakening of the ideological and political implications of the self-care philosophy, or should health education be restricted to purely technical issues and instructions for practical applications?

The answer to this question is not an easy one, since questions of ideology and politics are usually resolved by social processes and not by scientific or academic initiatives. Yet in this instance the magnitude of the problem is considerably restricted by the fact that the philosophy of health education is dominated by the need for a new conception of helping which will give individuals the qualifications they need to manage health questions in a responsible and effective manner and to take an active part in the prevention and therapy of illness. The way in which the problem is handled could very well emerge from the particular conditions of each case, while bearing always in mind the primary role played by the preferences and options of the specific public to which the programme is addressed.

On a more ideological level, self-care serves to influence the way in which problems and issues are defined. The health problems people face are basically personal ones that cannot be defined only in medical or social terms. By practising self-care, individuals or groups of people are able to establish alternative definitions of their condition. This ideological/practical tension is often presented as a dichotomy between changing the individual and changing the system. For this reason self-care often attracts professionals who want to alter the ways in which medical and social problems are defined and responded to.

Here, too, the attention of health care should be explicitly directed towards the development of these human powers—powers which, through emancipation and autonomous action, facilitate the realization of an emancipating ideal of liberty that contrasts with the alienating nature of our culture.[24]

AUTONOMY

Autonomy is a dominant value in the field of self-care. It involves respect for the individuality of others, recognition that people are defined by their values, and acceptance of their freedom to choose the way in which they live.

Two significant ethical issues focus on this crucial question. The first is concerned with whether health education programmes in self-care, when sponsored by the state, official institutions, or professional health services, could be considered as interference with the freedom of self-care practitioners and represent a real threat to their autonomy. The second is whether such interference could be justified by the benefits to be reaped, even when it takes the form of overt or covert paternalism.

It is argued, on the one hand, that self-care practitioners learn from each other's experience and from each other's knowledge. This knowledge comes from experience rather than from books or from the conventional 'authoritative' detached knowledge of the experts. That is why there is no reason for health professionals such as health educators to take part in the processes of self-care.[25]

It is also argued, on the other hand, that it is immoral and dangerous for man 'to play at being doctor' if no adequate techniques are available, and that technology needs to be developed by scientific research. Considerable effort would be required on the part of health educators, runs the argument, to teach people to use these newly developed technologies. In the framework of this rationale, justified paternalism claims that health educators are in a better position, because of superior information, to take the appropriate health protection measures than the individual.[26] Various criteria for justified paternalism are thus proposed in this direction, to take into account varying situations.[27,28]

It has also been suggested that paternalism to protect the public health is not only compatible with democratic values but that some of its aspects are essential for the defence of the common life and for promotion of a sense of community.

All these views rely principally on a utilitarian moral reasoning which takes the production of welfare or well-being as the criterion of right action. Only when respect for the patient's autonomy maximizes welfare is it morally required, and therefore paternalism is only misplaced when it reflects a miscalculation of benefits.[29]

It could thus be said that autonomy can have a more central position only in an entirely different frame of thought; within a moral theory which centres on action rather than on results, the precondition of agency will be fundamental. Using the above as a starting-point, within an action-orientated framework which takes account of the partial nature of human autonomy we can sketch patterns of reasoning which draw boundaries, in given contexts, between permissible and non-permissible forms of paternalism.

It should not be forgotten that one practitioner of self-care can indeed be expected to come to an informed and autonomous decision, but another may be too confused to understand adequately what the options are. Nor should we overlook the fact that some find the autonomous pursuit of goals a source rather of frustration and anxiety than of satisfaction. This is more often the case with discouraged patients, children, and the elderly, who may be unable, even when not wanting others to make their decisions for them, to make their own.

It is precisely awareness of the flexibility with which health education should move between respect for autonomy and the effectiveness of its contribution which is the best possible answer to this question. On the practical level, such an answer means that self-care education must develop out of the interests and preferences of lay people who are self-motivated to seek self-care skills. They must determine their 'curriculum' within the reasonable guidelines of the time and effect investments they wish to make and the utility of the skill itself.

CONCLUSIONS

A presentation of the most significant ethical issues involved in the implementation of self-care health education programmes makes it plain that the problems are both extensive and complex. I have tried in this Chapter to provide answers to some of these problems and to describe the fundamental aspects of others.

In conclusion, it should be emphasized that self-care is important and that health education can contribute to its development. It should also be stressed that if health education is to make an effective contribution without coming into conflict with fundamental values—whether those of self-care or of a more general nature—it must always be borne in mind that health is not the dominant value in life, that self-reliance is an expression of growth and human dignity, and that there is more than one medical culture.

If health education works on these principles it will be able to turn its attention to strengthening the natural resources of lay people as the basic resource for primary health care, designing specific programmes and techniques to promote the care-giving role of individuals, families, and other non-professional health care resources in the community. It will also be able, simultaneously, to minimize the ethical tensions which will arise between fundamental human values and existing needs.

REFERENCES

1. Bartlett, E.E. Educational self-help approaches in childhood asthma. *J Allergy Clin Immunol* 1983; **72**: 545–554.
2. Levin, L.S. The layperson as the primary health care practitioner. *Publ Hlth Rep* 1976; **91**: 2–6.
3. Litman, T.J. The family as a basic unit in health and medical care: a social behavioural overview. *Soc Sci Med* 1978; **5**: 495–519.
4. Mckinlay, J.B. and Kckinlay, S.M. The questionable contribution of medical measures to the decline of mortality in the twentieth century. *Hlth Soc* 1977; **55**: 405–428.
5. Kickbusch, I. and Hatch, S. A re-orientation of health care? In S. Hatch and I. Kickbusch (eds.). *Self-Help and Health in Europe*. Copenhagen: WHO, 1983.
6. Richardson, A. and Goodman, M. *Self-Help and Social Care: Mutual Aid Organisations in Practice*. London: Policy Studies Institute, 1983.
7. Katz, A.H. and Bender, E. *The Strength in Us: Self-Help Groups in the Modern World*. New York: Franklin Watts, 1976.
8. Schulte, B.M. Self-help and medical education. In S. Hatch and I. Kickbusch (eds.). *Self-Help and Health in Europe*. Copenhagen: WHO, 1983.
9. Grimso, A., Helgesen, G. and Borchgrevink, C. Short-term and long-term effects of lay groups on weight reduction. In S. Hatch, and I. Kickbusch (eds). *Self-Help and Health in Europe*. Copenhagen: WHO, 1983.
10. Matsuoka, K. Who teaches the patient? A team approach. *Diab Educ* 1984: 70–74.
11. Horowitz, L.G., Dillenberg, J. and Rattray, J. Self-care motivation: A model for primary preventive oral health behavior change. *J Sch Hlth* 1987; **57**: 114–118.
12. Nelson, E.C., Mchugo, G., Schnurr, P., *et al*. Medical self-care education for elders. A controlled trial to evaluate impact. *Am J Pub Hlth* 1984; **74**: 1357–1362.
13. McLendon, M.S., Fulk, C.H. and Starnes, D.C. Effectiveness of breast self-examination teaching to women of low socioeconomic class. *JOGN-Nurs* 1982; **11**: 7–10.
14. Buchinger, K. Self-help: a psychoanalyst's perspective. In S. Hatch and I. Kickbusch (eds.). *Self-Help and Health in Europe*. Copenhagen: WHO, 1983.
15. Maiman, L.A., Green, L.W., Gibson, G. and McKenzy, H.J. Education for self-treatment by adult asthmatics. *J Am Med Assoc* 1979; **241**: 1919–1923.
16. Greer, C. and Riessman, F. Better health care without more inflation. *Soc Pol* 1979; **10**: 2–3.
17. Stokes, B. Editorial. *Science*, 10 August, 1979.
18. Rolfi, J., Rozzini, R. and Trabucchi, M. Self-care education program in the elderly (letter to the editor). *J Am Med Assoc* 1984; **251**: 2929.

19. Owen, D. Medicine, morality, and the market (point of view). *Lancet* 1984; **i**: 30–31.
20. Fireman, P., Friday, G.A., Gira, C., Vierthaler, W.A., and Michaels, L. Teaching self-management skills to asthmatic children and their parents in an ambulatory care setting. *Pediatrics* 1981; **68**: 341–348.
21. Kemper, D.W. Self-care education: impact on HMO costs. *Med-Care* 1982; **20**: 710–718.
22. Barath, A. Hypertension clubs in Croatia. In S. Hatch and I. Kickbusch (eds.). *Self-Help and Health in Europe*. Copenhagen: WHO, 1983.
23. Drake, M. Self-help in the Soviet Union: the case of the deaf. In S. Hatch and I. Kickbusch (eds.). *Self-Help and Health in Europe*. Copenhagen: WHO, 1983.
24. Roszak, T. *Unfinished Animal, the Aquarian Frontier and the Evolution of Consciousness*. New York: Harper and Row, 1975.
25. Harberden, P. van and Lafaille, R. Over zelfhulpgroepen en professionals. *Anders* 1979; **2**: 817.
26. O'Connell, J. and Price, J. Ethical theories for promoting health through behaviours change. *J. School Hlth* 1983; **53**: 476–479.
27. Benjamin, M. and Curtis, J. *Ethics in Nursing*. New York: Oxford University Press, 1981.
28. Wikler, D. Coercive measures in health promotion: can they be justified? *Hlth Educ Mon* 1978; **6**: 223–241.
29. O'Neill, O. Paternalism and partial autonomy. *J Med Eth* 1984; **10**: 173–178.

CHAPTER 11

Health Education and the AIDS Epidemic

LEON EISENBERG

SUMMARY

This chapter begins with a review of what is known about the biology of AIDS. It next considers the social factors which influence disease transmission as well as public attitudes. After evaluating the methods available to control the epidemic, the Chapter considers the reasons for the limited success of public health measures thus far undertaken. It goes on to analyse the ethical debate on public health policy and concludes by emphasizing the need for a nationwide educational programme on AIDS, one which is responsive to the rights and obligations of citizens in a democratic society.

INTRODUCTION

To meet ethical standards, education about the acquired immunodeficiency syndrome (AIDS) should: (1) provide an accurate account of what is and is not known about the disease; (2) do so in language understandable to its intended audience; (3) offer guidelines which, if acted upon, will bring health benefits to individuals, families and communities; (4) and be so constructed as to promote the common good at the least cost to individual freedom.*

THE PUBLIC HEALTH PROBLEM POSED BY AIDS

As of July 1988, more than 100 000 cases of AIDS had been reported to the World Health Organization (WHO) from 138 countries; because under-reporting is extensive, WHO estimates the actual cumulative total at about 250 000 cases. By

---

*The chapters by Campbell on autonomy (Chapter 2), by Doxiadis and Garanis on health education for children (Chapter 8), and by Downie and Fyfe on school health education (Chapter 9) analyse ethical issues which are relevant to the argument set out in the present chapter.

Ethics in Health Education
Edited by S. Doxiadis. ©1990 John Wiley & Sons Ltd

extrapolation from fragmentary data on the population seroprevalence of antibodies to the human immunodeficiency virus (HIV), the number of infected persons has been estimated at between 5 and 10 million. Even at the lower estimate, about 1 million additional cases of AIDS can be expected to arise during the next five years from among those *already* infected by the virus.[1]

Geographically, there are three distinct patterns of HIV infection. In pattern I (predominant in North America, Western Europe, Australia, New Zealand, and urban areas of Latin America), sexual transmission occurs mainly among homosexual and bisexual men; transmission through blood results mainly from intravenous drug abuse. In pattern II (found in Sub-Saharan Africa and the Caribbean), sexual transmission is predominantly heterosexual; transmission through blood transfusions continues because programmes to screen out infected blood are not yet in place. Perinatal transmission to the newborn is a major problem; in some urban areas, 5–15% of pregnant women are infected by HIV. Pattern III (found in North Africa, the Middle East, Eastern Europe, Asia, and the Pacific) is characterized by relatively low rates of infection, primarily through exposure to imported blood and blood products or through sexual contact with travellers from pattern I and II areas.

Currently, neither a vaccine for the prevention of the disease nor a drug to cure it is available, nor is either foreseeable in the near future.[2] Available treatments are palliative. Hope of intercepting the epidemic rests upon the development of effective health education to change the behaviours which lead to disease transmission. Given the differences in prevalence and predominant modes of transmission, the focus of health education will necessarily vary from country to country.

THE BIOLOGY OF HIV INFECTION

AIDS was first recognized in 1981 because of the temporal conjunction of two unusual disease clusters in young men. The first was made up of cases of pneumonia caused by *Pneumocystis carinii*,[3] a fungus[4] which is pathogenic only in individuals debilitated by another disease; the second consisted of cases of Kaposi's sarcoma,[5] a rare skin cancer previously seen almost exclusively in elderly men.[6] The common feature of these two very different diseases is that 'opportunistic' infections (those which occur only in an immunologically compromised host) and secondary cancers had both been observed in patients receiving treatment with immunosuppressive drugs.[7] What was new was their occurrence in otherwise healthy young men without an ascertainable cause for suppression of the immune system. Cases fitting the epidemiological definition of AIDS were next discovered among intravenous drug addicts and recipients of blood transfusions of blood products.

It soon became evident that an epidemic was underway. Whereas the number of AIDS cases reported in the United States did not reach 800 until the end of 1982, it had risen to more than 7200 by the end of 1984, and had more than doubled again by the end of 1985. As of 28 November 1988, the cumulative United States total had risen to 79 389; the case fatality rate among patients diagnosed in the first three years of the epidemic and followed to the present exceeds 90%[8]. AIDS is occurring at disproportionately high rates among minority and poor populations.[9]

Contact tracing in the gay community, and from transfusion recipients to donors, implicated transmission of a hitherto unknown infectious particle through semen and blood.[10] By 1983, Montagnier's group at the Pasteur Institute in Paris[11] had identified, and Gallo's group at the National Institutes of Health in Washington[12] had confirmed, a retrovirus, now known as HIV, as the cause of the disease, and had developed antibody tests for the virus which made it possible to detect infection in asymptomatic individuals. Although a few reputable scientists still question HIV as the cause of AIDS,[13] the vast majority of active investigators regard the evidence for its causal role as clearly established.[14]

The determinants of the time lag between infection with the virus and the appearance of clinical disease and of the variability in its clinical manifestations are still not understood. A minority of HIV infected persons become immunosuppressed within the first year; about 25% will show overt AIDS and another 25% the AIDS-related complex (ARC) within five years of infection. As follow-up of infected individuals extends beyond five years, new clinical cases continue to arise; the ultimate proportion who will manifest clinical disease is still unknown.[15] The long silent period magnifies the public health problem. Because asymptomatic HIV infected persons are unaware of their status (and cannot be recognized by partners), unwitting disease transmission persists.

Although promising leads are under investigation, a fully effective treatment for AIDS or ARC continues to be elusive. In a 1987 randomized controlled clinical trial, zidovudine (azidothymidine, AZT) was shown to produce clinical benefit in patients during a 24 week treatment period; dose reduction or discontinuation was necessitated because of bone marrow toxicity in a number of patients.[16] As clinical research has continued, zidovudine's initial benefits appear not to be sustainable. Dournon and colleagues [17] have reported, in a consecutive series of 365 treated patients, that most clinical and laboratory indices had reverted to their initial values by six months. Recombinant interferon-alpha has shown promising results in AIDS-related Kaposi's sarcoma, with a major beneficial response in 12 of 26 patients in one trial[18] and eight of 21 in a second.[19] Phase I studies of zidovudine and interferon-alpha combined therapy are currently underway, as are trials with other putative therapeutic agents.

Developing a vaccine against HIV infection has proved to be a difficult task because of the characteristics of the virus and the nature of the host response. To begin with, there is extensive genetic variation among virus isolates; indeed, the virus continues to mutate within the human host so that multiple new variants appear during the course of infection.[20] This extraordinary mutability (at a rate estimated to be a million times that of eukaryotic DNA genomes) may arise from high error rates in the replication of the retroviral genome because of the low fidelity of HIV encoded reverse transcriptase.[21,22] Second, the virus integrates its genetic code into the genome of cells in the human host once infection occurs; thus, infection is lifelong. Third, although infection results in antibody production, anti-HIV antibodies are relatively ineffective in neutralizing the virus. Fourth, there is still no satisfactory animal laboratory model for AIDS.[23]

Even after promising vaccines have been fabricated in the laboratory and have been shown to be immunogenic and non-toxic in human volunteers, there are formidable obstacles in the way of controlled epidemiological trials. Because of the long latent period between infection and the appearance of clinical disease, trials will require not less than three to five years to determine whether the vaccine confers effective protection. Recipients of a trial vaccine, once they seroconvert, will need special means of identification to protect them from being mislabelled as infected. To the extent that AIDS education—obviously a public health priority and an ethical obligation to the volunteer participants—succeeds in reducing high risk behaviour in both the experimental and the 'placebo' vaccine subjects, it will diminish the likelihood of demonstrating vaccine potency, even if it is present.

THE SOCIAL DIMENSIONS OF HIV INFECTION

Because AIDS was first recognized in the United States among male homosexuals and, shortly thereafter, among intravenous drug abusers, political conservatives as well as fundamentalist religious leaders interpreted the disease as the physical embodiment of the sufferer's moral defilement. They did not disguise their grim satisfaction at what they considered to be the wages of sin,[24] just as, earlier in the century, syphilis had been regarded as a moral problem rather than as a disease warranting a public health response.[25] Yet, vulnerability to AIDS does not result from homosexuality per se, but from unprotected intercourse with an infected partner. Nor does AIDS result from drug abuse as such. High rates of infection among intravenous drug users stem, not from drugs, but from sharing contaminated drug equipment.

Public panic was conjoined with moral opprobrium when the disease spread to 'innocent victims'—recipients of blood transfusions,[26] haemophiliacs dependent on donor-derived factor VIII,[27] female sexual partners of infected men,[28] babies born to infected mothers,[29] women impregnated by artificial insemination,[30] and health care workers accidentally punctured by needles.[31] The reassurance the general public had taken from the apparently low rate of heterosexual transmission eroded with the recognition of almost equal male/female sex ratios in sub-Saharan Africa. Public demand for action grew. Government authorities were forced to face issues they had been trying to avoid because of their inability to satisfy the claims of all constituencies.

Cooperation between nations was impeded by a dispute about the origins of the disease. African seroprevalence data and the discovery of a simian immunodeficiency virus (SIV) endemic among green monkeys led to speculation that SIV was the viral precursor for HIV. Recently reported nucleotide sequence data on SIV[32] and HIV variants[33] make SIV an unlikely source for HIV. However, the damage had been done. The hypothesis of an African origin of AIDS was bitterly resented by Africans who took this as yet another example of colonial mentality. The dispute contributed to a delay in acknowledging the extent of the public health problem in Africa. Although the reasons for the epidemiological differences between pattern I and pattern II countries are not entirely clear, they are likely to have arisen from accidents of history and culturally determined differences in behaviour. In the United States, HIV infection apparently began first among a subset of the homosexual male community.[34] Rapid spread was the tragic but inevitable result of patterns of sexual behaviour which had become prevalent in the fast lane of the gay community in the 1960s and 1970s—sexual congress with multiple and constantly changing partners in gay establishments (bars, bath houses, and the back rooms of cinemas). It is likely that vulnerability to HIV was enhanced by the high prevalence of other sexually transmitted disease (STDs) in this subpopulation. Homosexual intravenous drug users unwittingly introduced HIV into the addict population. There it spread very rapidly among users sharing equipment in 'shooting galleries' (underground establishments renting space and equipment to use in shooting up and sometimes providing 'street doctors' expert in needling collapsed veins). AIDS in women, who account for less than one case in 10 in the United States, results primarily from drug abuse and sexual intercourse with bisexual men or male addicts or both.

In Africa, in contrast, transmission through homosexual intercourse and intravenous drug use is far less common. There, spread has been fostered by multiple heterosexual partners, a high prevalence of other STDs,[35] widespread female prostitution in urban centres consequent upon massive rural outmigration, and the transfusion of infected blood, all leading to the nearly 1:1 male/female ratio.[36]

INTERRUPTING HIV TRANSMISSION

The facts thus far established about how HIV is, and is not, transmitted from one person to another provide the scientific foundation for control measures. The three principal modes of transmission are (1) by sexual intercourse with an infected partner; (2) by infected blood and blood products, and (3) by placental passage from infected mother to fetus. HIV is *not* transmitted through casual or even intimate non-sexual interpersonal contacts within families, in the workplace, or at school.[37] Whether it can be transmitted by orogenital contact, by deep kissing, or breast feeding is not known.

Changes in the preparation of factor VIII and other blood products have made those products entirely safe for use. Antibody screening of donated blood has markedly, though not entirely, reduced the risk of HIV transmission by transfusion wherever screening has been introduced; risk persists, however, because of the 30–90-day time window between the onset of HIV infection and the production of antibodies detectable by current screening measures.[38] Systematic screening of semen donors (freezing the semen until repeat HIV antibody testing on donors initially and after six months has established its safety) has minimized the risk associated with artificial insemination. Infectious disease precautions have limited, though not abolished, the relatively low risk for health care workers.[31] There are, however, no fully effective technological fixes for the two most common modes of HIV transmission, sexual intercourse (homosexual or heterosexual) and intravenous drug use, and none at all for perinatal transmission, other than aborting the fetus because of a 40-to 50% risk of infection.

Although the use of latex condoms (which do not allow HIV to pass the physical barrier they interpose between penis and vagina) plus virucidal spermicides (which contain nonoxynol 9) reduces risk,[39] condoms are not fail-safe as is evident from their imperfect record as contraceptives; they may be defective in manufacture, they may be torn or slip off during use, and they must be properly applied before each episode of intercourse. Some men are reluctant to use condoms on the grounds that they diminish pleasure in the sexual act, and others because they are contraceptives; in many countries, condoms are not readily accessible.

With intravenous drug use, the danger is inherent in the use of shared paraphernalia (needles and syringes). The virus is transmitted from infected to uninfected persons by means of the residual blood in the apparatus when it is passed from one individual to another. The interruption of intravenous drug use (the obviously preferable public health solution—were it possible) or the use of sterile needles and syringes will abolish this mode of transmission. Alternatively, because HIV is a relatively fragile virus, the proper use of a diluted solution of household bleach to clean equipment between use can reduce the likelihood of transmission.

THE LEVEL OF PUBLIC KNOWLEDGE

In view of the extensive media coverage given to the AIDS epidemic in industrialized (pattern I) countries, is there a need for additional health information? Sequential public opinion polls since 1983 reveal growing awareness of AIDS, the risk it poses to health, and some of the facts about infectivity; they also demonstrate that misinformation persists.[40] The National Health Interview Survey[41] interviews a probability sample of the United States civilian non-institutionalized population at regular intervals. A survey of some 3100 persons on knowledge and attitudes about AIDS in September 1987 revealed that almost all had heard of AIDS; 98% knew it to be fatal, 95% believed that it could be transmitted by sexual intercourse, 76% that it was caused by a virus, 68% that it could be transmitted by transfusion. However, substantial numbers were grossly misinformed. One-third or more of the respondents thought it was definitely or probably true that AIDS could be contracted by sharing eating utensils, eating in a restaurant where the cook had AIDS, being coughed or sneezed upon by a person with AIDS, using public toilets, or being bitten by insects! One-quarter considered that the disease could be acquired by *donating* blood and one-sixth by working near, shaking hands with, or going to school with, a person with AIDS. Whereas 82% knew condoms could prevent transmission, 13% believed diaphragms to be effective as well.

Anonymous questionnaires distributed to some 600 students at an eastern United States university[42] showed them to be more knowledgeable than the general public; nonetheless, one-eighth of the students were concerned about 'catching' AIDS in public toilets, one-quarter believed that infected individuals should not be allowed to live in dormitories, and one-eighth that they should not be allowed to attend classes. Less than 20% of the students who reported having multiple sexual partners, whether homosexual or heterosexual, had changed their sexual behaviour because of the danger of HIV infection. In a current San Francisco study[43] of 500 sexually active teenagers, only 2% of the boys and 8% of the girls used condoms consistently; no less disturbing was the finding that 30% engaged in unprotected anal intercourse, the sexual behaviour most closely associated with HIV transmission in the United States.

A public opinion survey of social perception of AIDS[44] in France revealed that 37% continue to believe AIDS can be transmitted by blood donation, and 10% by mosquito bites, by drinking from a patient's glass, or in public lavatories. Those who were the least informed were the most likely to favour mandatory screening for HIV infection and isolation of AIDS patients (as was true in the United States university study).

The situation is somewhat different but still far from satisfactory among the two populations in western countries at greatest risk: sexually active homosexuals and intravenous drug addicts. Among selected (that is, middle class, highly educated, and self-declared) American gay populations, AIDS knowledge is greater and reported reduction in high risk behaviour is more extensive.[45,46] In parallel, there has been a decline in rates of HIV seroconversion and in the prevalence of other STDs among such groups. These changes likely reflect the enormous emotional and social impact AIDS has had on the organized gay community.[47,48] Nonetheless, a significant proportion continue to engage in behaviours they report they know place them at high risk for infection. Moreover, the recently reported increase in rates for syphilis in the United States,[49] primarily among Blacks and Hispanics, reflects (1) the failure of current efforts to reach minority populations and (2) the diversion of resources from other STD control programmes to support AIDS control efforts. Among intravenous drug addicts, sharing equipment is widely known to be dangerous. An illegal market in allegedly sterile needles has grown in New York City; yet sharing continues to be the modal behaviour pattern.[9]

Thus, there is an urgent need, not only for more, but for more effective, health education.

BARRIERS TO AIDS EDUCATION

AIDS education faces formidable obstacles. Stating information clearly and disseminating it widely in language understandable to target populations are necessary, but not sufficient. Individuals at risk must be motivated to change their actions and must have the skills to do so; to maintain safer behaviours, continuous social reinforcement is necessary. When the established behaviours involve sexual practices and drug use, change is predictably difficult to effect.[50] For almost two decades, unprotected sexual intercourse has been the norm among American teenagers, evident in the fact that the United States has the highest teenage pregnancy rates—although it does not have the highest rates of premarital intercourse—among industrialized nations.[51] As to intravenous drug use, not only is needle sharing part of its subculture, but addicts made desperate by withdrawal will use whatever equipment they can find. Long-term disease prevention from either mode of transmission demands sustained behaviour change (in contrast to the one time decision to be vaccinated without having to change the rest of one's behavioural repertoire).

In face of the powerful social and cultural forces which maintain high-risk behaviour, the federal commitment to AIDS education can only be called paltry. In 1986, the Institute of Medicine/National Academy of Sciences[52] called for annual expenditures of a billion dollars for AIDS education and related public health measures by 1990. The allocation did not reach $315 million until 1988; the budget proposed by the administration for 1989 was only $400 million. The Presidential Commission on AIDS, notwithstanding its appointment by the incumbent administration, severely criticized the inadequacy of the federal effort and called for a far more ambitious undertaking.[53]

The effectiveness of education has been further compromised by reluctance to use explicit terminology. In the first years of the epidemic, American media employed the term 'bodily fluids' as a euphemism for semen or blood. The ambiguous language added to public panic because it was interpreted to include saliva, sweat, and tears. Even the instructions inserted in commercial condom packages require the reading level of a high school graduate for full comprehension, making the instructions virtually useless for those in most need of them.[54]

ETHICAL ISSUES IN RELATION TO RISK REDUCTION

The United States effort to control HIV infection has been bedevilled by strongly held differences about what is and is not morally acceptable in public policy. Although ours is a democracy with a constitutionally prescribed separation between church and state, the cultural and ethnic heterogeneity of our population has resulted in divergent religious and secular viewpoints. Fashioning coherent public policy out of the claims of competing constituencies represents an as yet unsolved political challenge.

The public debate can be most clearly epitomized by contrasting two opposing camps: public health advocates versus moralizers. The former adopt a pragmatic, consequentialist position, one that can be termed ethical realism; the latter base themselves on religious fundamentalism and claim they are 'the moral majority' in the United States. Their morality has been challenged; public opinion polls have demonstrated that they are far from the majority. It is true that some physicians adopt a moralizing stance and some religious leaders accept the urgency of pragmatic measures at the same time that they advocate moral suasion. Yet, this antithesis conveys the essence of the controversy. Each position reflects implicit as well as explicit social values about sexuality, medicine and disease.

The public health position finds no moral meaning in disease phenomenology. Its goal is the reduction of morbidity and mortality to the minimum achievable by existing means. Advocates specify their goals in operational terms and rest their case on empirical evaluation. The question they ask is: does a given measure in fact reduce disease transmission? Their position was eloquently stated by Thomas Sydenham[55] in 1673 when he defended his studies of venereal disease treatment against the charge that they contributed to immorality by removing 'the fear of future trouble' which 'terrifies the unchaste':

'If we reject all cases of affliction which the improvidence of human beings has brought upon themselves, there will be but little room left for the exercise of mutual love and charity. God alone punishes. We, as best we can, must relieve . . . Hence I will state what I have observed and tried in the disease in question; and that not with the view of making men's minds more immoral, but for the sake of making their bodies sounder. This is the business of the physician.'

For the moralizers, the prevention of disease, though desirable in itself, is secondary in value to more fundamental moral precepts about the good life. In the eyes of many fundamentalists, disease itself plays a role in the moral order of the world. Behaviourally transmitted diseases serve a moral function in so far as fear of contracting them encourages continence. To remove that fear by medical means is to encourage immorality. Thus, Norman Podhoretz[56] a spokesman for the New Right, condemned political leaders who called for a crash programme to develop an AIDS vaccine: 'Are they aware,' he asked, 'that in the name of compassion they are giving social sanction to what can only be described as brutish degradation?'

Earlier in this century, when syphilis was epidemic, the social hygiene movement had insisted that the best way to prevent infection was by adherence to an ethic that restricted sexual relationships to marriage, a goal that was to be achieved through education to encourage abstinence and the repression of prostitution.[57] Measures to prevent syphilis or to treat it, by making sex safer, could only encourage promiscuity. Indeed, a leading American dermatologist,[58] after the remarkable success of penicillin in treating syphilis, felt impelled to write:

'It is a reasonable question, whether by eliminating disease, without commensurate attention to the development of human idealism, self control, and responsibility in sexual life, we are not bringing mankind to its fall instead of its fulfillment.'

These contrasting views have been widely voiced in the years since the magnitude of the AIDS epidemic became apparent. They lead to sharply different conclusions about disease containment.

The position of the religious right on homosexuality is based on biblical injunctions interpreted as condemning such behaviour. Whatever his desires and however they arise, the homosexual is deemed capable of the moral choice to renounce his impulses. If he opts for celibacy, he can be forgiven; if he continues on his path, he has rejected salvation. To instruct a sinner on how to maintain his health while continuing to sin is to foster immoral behaviour. To educate children about homosexuality except to condemn it is to place temptation in their way. The only moral way, they contend, indeed, the most effective way, to limit the spread of disease among homosexuals is by demanding that they abandon their 'style of life.' Because, in this view, homosexual behaviour is a wilful choice, AIDS becomes a self-inflicted disease.

The consequentialist position places health outcomes first. Whether the genesis of homosexuality is taken to be biologically determined, socially shaped, or freely chosen is irrelevant; the central facts are its occurrence and the health risks associated with it. The public health goal is education about risk reduction. To do so effectively requires that homosexuals be treated with respect as fellow human beings. The self-proclaimed moralist's fear that telling adolescents the facts about homosexuality will seduce them is a fear without data to support it. Providing all citizens with the facts about disease transmission in order to enable them to modify their behaviour accordingly is the fundamental ethos of the realist.

The moralizer believes that premarital and extramarital sex are sins to be condemned. Although the preservation of life is a desideratum, it is secondary in importance to living a moral life. Adherence to morality, so defined, will in itself obviate sexually transmitted diseases. Sex education is the primary responsibility of family and church. If it is to be permitted in schools, moral context must take precedence over physiology. Those who believe that intercourse is allowable only when it permits procreation regard instruction about condoms as unacceptable; condoms are contraceptives even if they are ostensibly used for disease prevention.

The consequentialist position on sexuality begins with the recognition that premarital experimentation is widespread in contemporary society. Whether it be taken to be a component of normal sexual development or a deviation from mature sexuality, it will not be changed by exhortation. Because ignorance about sex not only fails to delay sexual expression but transmutes it into a high risk activity, public health advocates focus on what is feasible; namely, the provision of full information about how disease transmission can be minimized and ready access to condoms to increase their use when intercourse does occur.

Ethical realists no less than moralizers view intravenous drug abuse as inherently self-destructive. Where the two differ is in the stance they take on how it can be controlled and on measures to limit the disease transmission associated with it. Whereas the medical viewpoint is compatible with a variety of control measures extending from strict legal interdiction through methadone maintenance to drug-free treatment programmes (to the extent their effectiveness is supported by empirical evidence), the moralizer accepts only strict interdiction and rejects methadone maintenance as substituting addiction to one drug for another. There is a further contrast. Those who focus on health outcomes point to the obvious failure of law enforcement to control the drug trade, the unwillingness of many addicts to accept treatment, and the high recidivism rate among those addicts who do enter treatment programmes. In view of these demonstrable facts, although consequentialists support augmented treatment efforts, they simultaneously advocate educating addicts about health risks and making sterile injection equipment available in order to minimize disease transmission. To the religious moralizer, making drug use safer is to condone it and thus contribute to its prevalence. No less dismayed by the spread of AIDS, particularly when it is transmitted to unknowing spouses and to offspring, they insist that stricter law enforcement and stronger penalties are the appropriate public response.

Premarital sexual continence, sexual fidelity in marriage, and cessation of intravenous drug abuse—the propositions put forth by the moralizers—would indeed halt HIV transmission. Because none of these goals has even the most remote chance of being attained, public health advocates promote pragmatic policies, admittedly partial and imperfect, to control disease. They cite the modest but persuasive evidence for effectiveness. That evidence is dismissed by the religious right as irrelevant to what matters most: public morality. The result of the controversy has been to require compromise in, but not to halt, education campaigns.

SCIENCE, HUMAN RIGHTS, AND AIDS POLICY

To attain the goal of interrupting disease transmission, AIDS education must increase public understanding of the technical questions and the human rights issues which underlie public policy. This is a formidable challenge. Public education about the scientific method is lamentably inadequate; scepticism about science and scientists is widespread.[24] Few understand that 'safety' can never be absolute and that 'risk' is always relative. Research on the factors influencing choice in the face of uncertainty has shown that the way the alternatives are presented can influence subjective assessment even when the two presentations are mathematically equivalent.[59]

In the debate about mandatory screening for HIV infection, the dispute is between those who assert a public 'right to know' and who claim that mandatory testing is necessary to prevent 'ignorant transmission' of the virus; and those who give greater weight to individual rights and assert on pragmatic grounds that voluntary testing is far more likely to succeed.

Advocates of mandatory testing allege that it would benefit the community at large by providing accurate epidemiological data and by opening avenues (including quarantine) to control the behaviour of infected individuals. The victims themselves, they contend, would benefit from the counselling that would be provided and by being informed of (or even required by law to accept) such treatment measures as are available at a given time. Advocates differ as to how far they would carry mandatory HIV testing. Some insist it be universal, others would make it a condition for marriage licensure and hospital admission, still others would limit its application to individuals known to be engaging in high risk behaviour.

Opponents dispute these claims on both civil libertarian and pragmatic grounds. To begin with, compulsory testing violates the right of privacy. Because of the social stigma associated with HIV infection, those identified as seropositive would be exposed to the risk of losing jobs, being turned out of rented apartments, being barred from school, being denied health and life insurance, and being rejected by family and friends, events that continue to be everyday occurrences. Confidentiality of medical information is easier to promise than to guarantee. Although opponents of mandatory testing acknowledge the importance of better epidemiological data, they contend that such information can be gathered by anonymous testing in hospitals, clinics, and volunteer test sites. The failure to make assurance of confidentiality credible by additional legal protection[53] currently impairs voluntary test programmes.

In a recent Oregon study[60] which compared an anonymous test site with one that required names but promised confidentiality, usage doubled at the anonymous site; many more infected persons obtained counselling. The Japanese Ministry of Health and Welfare has proposed an 'AIDS Prevention Bill' which mandates reporting HIV carriers to prefectural authorities. To examine the effects of official notification upon willingness to be tested, Ohi and colleagues[61] questioned large groups of Japanese workers, students, male homosexuals, and female prostitutes on their willingness to accept testing under such a circumstance. Their findings indicate a sizeable decline in compliance were the bill to become law, especially among the at-risk groups (homosexuals and prostitutes). They conclude that 'the effect of the bill might be the opposite of what is intended.'

Mandatory HIV testing as a requirement for employment in occupations where public safety is at stake—for example, mass transportation—has been proposed in several countries. Although screening is rationalized as preventing the potential danger posed by an impaired airline pilot or air traffic controller, it is also clear that industry has a major financial stake in screening out new workers at risk for illness or premature death in order to avoid low returns on the investment in job training and higher insurance costs. These facts do not in themselves gainsay the importance of examining implications for public safety, but do suggest caution in accepting such claims at face value. What is the evidence?

Autopsy data have revealed that extensive infection of the central nervous system is frequent in advanced stages of AIDS; such patients exhibit severe cognitive and emotional neuropsychiatric disorders termed the AIDS dementia complex (ADC).[62] ADC can appear well before the terminal stages of AIDS,[63] but is rare in the absence of other clinical signs and symptoms.[64] In a carefully controlled study of cognitive function in a cohort of gay volunteers, persons who were evaluated before and after their HIV serostatus was determined, Kessler and colleagues[65] found no significant differences between seropositive and seronegative subjects *before* they knew their status; however, psychometric test performance of seropositive individuals declined significantly *after* they had been informed; that is, observed post-test deterioration in HIV positive individuals resulted from psychosocial stress rather than HIV infection per se.

Although negative findings even in a relatively large cohort cannot completely exclude the possibility of rare instances of cognitive impairment in seropositive but otherwise clinically well individuals, this risk must be assessed in relation to other far more common hazards; for example, impairment resulting from alcohol or illicit drugs,[66] minor tranquillizers,[67] disruption of circadian rhythm caused by journeys across multiple time zones,[68] and other diseases.[69,70]

Protecting public safety in mass transport is best assured by efforts to develop more sensitive methods for early detection of significant deterioration of function, whatever its cause.[71,72] Thus, the World Health Organization (WHO) Global Programme on AIDS Consultation on the Neuropsychiatric Aspects of HIV Infection concluded that there is *at present* 'no evidence for an increase of clinically significant neuropsychiatric abnormalities' in *otherwise asymptomatic* HIV seropositive persons and 'no justification for...screening as a strategy.'[73]

Mandatory testing involves disproportionate costs for meagre results. The predictive value of a positive finding on a screening test depends not only on the accuracy of the method but also on the prevalence of the disease in the population being tested. The nature of the problem can be illustrated by the following two examples. Though they are 'thought experiments', they are based on realistic field conditions. In the first, screening is applied to a population with low seroprevalence, in the second, to one with a very high rate.

Consider the results when a screening test, the enzyme immunoassay (EIA) is applied to 100 000 persons with a true seroprevalence of 0.5% (approximately that estimated for the United States as a whole). When performed under optimal conditions, the EIA is remarkably accurate. It has a sensitivity (the proportion of infected persons who test positive) of about 98% and a specificity (the proportion of *un*infected persons who test negative) of somewhat better than 99%. Yet, when the EIA for HIV antibodies is applied to this study population, it will generate the findings presented in Table 1.

The test will yield 995 false positives (that is, a positive result in the absence of infection) for the 490 true positives it identified, a FP/TP ratio of more than 2 to 1! The predictive power of a positive test would be 33%. Almost 1000 persons

Table 1   Findings of a screening test (EIA for HIV antibodies) applied to 100 000 individuals with a true seroprevalence of 0.5%

	HIV infection	No HIV infection	Total
EIA positive	490	995	1 485
EIA negative	10	98 505	98 515
Total	500	99 500	100 000

(1% of the population tested) would be exposed to the devastating consequences of being told they are infected by HIV, when in fact they are not. Clearly, it would be imperative to carry out confirmatory tests by the closest there is to a gold standard, the Western blot (WB). On prescreened sera, the WB has a sensitivity of 92% and a specificity of 95%. If it were applied to EIA test positive sera (the negatives, including 10 false negatives, not being subject to retest), the findings would be those in Table 2.

The final result is now 451 true positives detected, 49 missed, and 50 false positives still misidentified.

If the EIA were to be applied to a population of 100 000 with a true seroprevalence of 50% (a rate approximating to that among sexually active San Francisco gays and intravenous drug addict subpopulations in Newark and New York City), the reliability of positive test findings would change dramatically. This situation is illustrated in Table 3.

Testing would yield one false positive for each 98 true positives. The predictive power of a positive test would be 99%. There would, of course, still be the necessity for WB confirmatory testing (Table 4).

Table 2   Findings of a confirmatory test (Western blot) applied to EIA test-positive sera from population in Table 1

	HIV infection	No HIV infection	Total
WB positive	451	50	501
WB negative	39	945	984
Not tested	10	98 505	98 515
Total	500	99 900	100 000

Table 3   Findings of a screening test (EIA for HIV antibodies) applied to a population of 100 000 with a true seroprevalence of 50%

	HIV infection	No HIV infection	Total
EIA positive	49 000	500	49 500
EIA negative	1 000	49 500	50 500
Total	50 000	50 000	100 000

Table 4   Findings of a confirmatory test (Western blot) applied to EIA test-positive sera from population in Table 3

	HIV infection	No HIV infection	Total
WB positive	45 080	25	45 105
WB negative	3 920	475	4 395
Not tested	1 000	49 500	50 500
Total	50 000	50 000	100 000

The net result would be 45 080 true positives identified at the cost of 3920 missed (7.8%) but only 25 persons out of the original population (0.025%) falsely labelled as infected. Despite the quite extraordinary accuracy of these tests (far beyond that of most tests in common use), both false negative and false positive results are inescapable—with all the human costs they entail.

Cleary and colleagues[74] undertook a careful quantitative analysis of the findings to be expected if mandatory premarital screening were to be enforced in the United States. Their calculations were more precise than those exemplified in the preceding tables because they took into account known variations in seropositivity by gender and age and more precise figures for EIA and WB sensitivity and specificity. Premarital screening would detect fewer than 0.1% of those tested as HIV infected, would mislabel more than 450 (100 as false negative and 350 as false positive) and would entail the expenditure of well over $100 million. If mandatory testing were to be instituted nationwide, the fiscal costs and negative social consequences would be more than one hundred fold greater. The funds expended would yield far greater benefits if applied to public education and voluntary testing. Experience in one state (Illinois) with a mandatory testing programme has led even its proponents to consider repeal of the legislation: state marriage rates dropped (many couples went to neighbouring states to escape the requirement); test facilities were swamped; very few new cases were uncovered.[75,76] Among the first 45 000 persons tested, five were positive; the cost for each identified case of HIV infection was about $715 000![77]

The WHO Global Programme on AIDS convened a meeting of international experts to consider criteria for HIV screening programmes in May 1987.[78] The participants concluded that:

'readily accessible counselling and testing for antibody to HIV, provided on a voluntary basis, are more likely to result in behaviour changes that contribute to the public health goal of reducing spread of HIV than are mandatory screening initiatives ... Epidemiological surveillance data can be obtained, as needed, by methods that do not compromise human rights. The complexity of logistic, technical, personal, social, legal and ethical issues generated by mandatory screening of targeted populations must be recognized.'

Data on HIV seroprevalence in the population can be obtained without putting confidentiality at risk and without depending upon voluntary assent by testing blood specimens obtained for routine medical uses after removing identifying personal information. Such studies are most easily done in hospitals or outpatient clinics by screening residual blood in specimens taken for other purposes. From an epidemiological standpoint, the findings will not be representative of a random population sample, since the test sera derive from persons who are seeking medical care. However, for particular purposes, testing anonymous specimens can be fully informative; for example, in bloods drawn from pregnant women at term since virtually all urban births are delivered in hospital. Such data present accurately the status of the population served by specific hospitals[79,80].

Although anonymous testing of residual blood specimens does not jeopardize confidentiality, the procedure has been criticized on the grounds that a patient's blood can not ethically be used for any purpose other than that specified when the patient agreed to have it drawn. This objection has not been persuasive to Institutional Review Boards when they have been asked to rule on the matter; the residual blood would otherwise simply be discarded as waste matter; testing provides information of use to the community (and, therefore, to the patient as a member of the community). The method does carry a distinct liability: once personal identifiers have been removed from blood specimens, there is no way to notify seropositive persons of their status.

Even if one agrees that voluntary testing and anonymous sampling are preferable to mandatory screening under present circumstances, would the same judgment be warranted (a) if test error were to be significantly reduced and (b) if means to eliminate infectivity were to become available at some time in the future? Let us consider each in turn.

Error rates can be—and are being—minimized by more exacting confirmatory Western blot standards.[81] New test methods are under development in research laboratories. They are based upon the use of the polymerase chain reaction to amplify specific segments of the HIV genome[82] and permit direct detection of infection independent of antibody response.[83,84] However, reduction of test error rates alone does not suffice to establish the public health utility of mass screening, as Weiss and Thier[85] have shown in an editorial pointedly entitled: 'HIV testing is the answer—what's the question?' In the absence of a cure for AIDS, the purpose of testing is to reduce transmission by changing the behaviour of infected persons. Evidence of behaviour change among individuals who choose to be tested on a voluntary basis cannot be generalized to those who are given information they have not sought.

The New York Blood Bank urges donors not to give blood for transfusion if they have engaged in high risk behaviour; it provides a confidential form on which potential donors can designate their blood 'for studies only' if they are in a risk category. Nonetheless, such individuals continue to give blood for transfusion.[86] When notified of their seropositivity and reinterviewed, 90% acknowledged that they fell into a risk class (though only 10% 'believed' they would test positive). Moreover, even after counselling, some infected persons persist in high risk behaviours.[87] In the absence of more effective means of bringing about behaviour change among those notified of their serostatus, improved precision in screening will not in itself justify mandatory screening.

Suppose, however, that research yields a drug capable of suppressing infection and, more to the point of the present discussion, of abolishing infectivity. Under such a circumstance, identifying infected persons through screening would not only make possible direct benefit to them but also provide the means to halt the spread of infection in the community. Mandatory screening would then appear in a new light. While it seems probable that almost all seropositive persons would seek treatment in view of their almost inevitable progression to severe disease, debate about public policy would soon shift to the question of mandatory treatment for those who refused to accept it voluntarily and thus continued to put others in jeopardy. These are public health precedents for compulsory treatment: in many jurisdictions, individuals with active tuberculosis who refuse care can be confined to sanatoria by court order. Given the far greater lethality of AIDS, one can anticipate that the vast majority of the public would support mandatory screening and mandatory treatment, were such a drug to become available.

The matter will almost certainly not be so simple from a medical standpoint as the preceding discussion suggests. It is highly unlikely that an agent will be discovered that is both completely effective in suppressing infectivity and altogether without toxicity; thus far, every promising drug has had major side-effects. However persuasive the argument to be constructed for compulsory treatment by a 'fully effective' and 'completely benign' drug, the less certain its therapeutic potential and the greater its toxicity, the more difficult will be the resolution of the trade-off between individual autonomy and the community interest in interdicting the epidemic.

WHAT IS TO BE DONE?

Despite the absence of a vaccine capable of preventing HIV infection or a treatment able to cure it, what is known about its modes of transmission make control of the HIV epidemic a feasible goal, but only if citizens are effectively informed about what is (and is not) known and what they can do individually and collectively to promote health among those currently well and to provide care for those who have already been infected. Citizens need to understand not only what modifications they need to make in their own behaviour as individuals but must also be thoroughly familiar with the issues at stake in formulating public health policy.

There can be no question of withholding facts (such as the inability to assure complete safety of the blood supply), but scientific presentations and media reports on those presentations should take care to put them in context—that is, compare the risk of infection from transfusion with the hazard of refusing it when it is medically necessary. The specificity of the information provided and the explicitness of the language by which it is transmitted should be tailored to the groups at whom the campaign is targeted. Thus, the details of gay sex behaviour and 'eroticizing' safe sex will be of low relevance for the general population but crucial in enabling homosexuals to avoid disease. A level of explicitness which may be deemed offensive to the population at large is nevertheless essential for reaching specific groups; it can be provided through channels other than mass madia. Gay self-help groups have prepared pamphlets, made video tapes, and organized group discussions for their own constituencies. Detached street workers, often former drug addicts employed by health departments, have been able to contact intravenous drug users who need graphic demonstration on how to sterilize equipment. The credibility of the individuals providing the information is a crucial determinant of whether it will be believed.[88]

The success[45,46] of safe sex education programmes produced and sponsored by gay organizations has been nothing short of remarkable: annualized seroconversion rates in probability samples of homosexual men in San Francisco have fallen from 18.4% before 1984 to 4.2% in 1986 and to 0.7% in the second half of 1987![89] But this has been limited to the primarily middle class, educated, mostly white men who openly acknowledge a gay self-identification. There is little evidence the message reaches closet gays, members of ethnic minority groups, and bisexuals who do not identify themselves as homosexual. The complexity of the issue is illustrated by Brazilian culture, where the ideology of machismo is prominent. The notion of a gay identity is a recent import from North America and is applied only to those who are the passive or recipient partners in homosexual pairs.[90] Men who are the active or masculine partners (that is, those who insert the phallus) in homosexual intercourse are by definition not gay, a category which they regard as invidious. Thus, were HIV educational efforts to be directed at 'gays' in Brazil, they would necessarily fail to reach key links in the disease transmission chain.

AIDS education for addicts has hardly begun and is still not routinely incorporated into drug treatment programmes. There has been a two-and-a-half-fold increase in deaths among intravenous drug users in New York City coincident with the AIDS epidemic, despite no discernible change in the number of users. About one-third of the excess deaths have been directly attributed to AIDS. However, Stoneburner and colleagues[91] conclude that AIDS accounts for many more of the excess deaths because autopsy data reveal the presence of infections and other diseases associated with HIV infection. Because such deaths occur disproportionately among black and Hispanic intravenous drug users, current data underestimate the impact of AIDS in minority communities. Clearly, such individuals are not being reached by drug treatment programmes and by education about the importance of clean works.

The limited success associated with health education for the population at large makes evident the need for experimentation with new approaches. As Warwick and colleagues[92] point out, broadcasting the 'scientific facts' to passive recipients is insufficient to produce change in health related behaviours. Educational planning must begin by discovering through ethnographic methods what it is particular groups (for example, teenagers) believe and what worries them in order to design interactive formats to promote behaviour change. Enthusiasm and good intentions cannot substitute for evidence of effectiveness. The imperative is for a major commitment to evaluation research, thus far sadly lacking.

In late May 1988, at a cost of $17.4 million, 106 million copies of the Surgeon General's brochure *Understanding AIDS* were distributed to all American households, post office box holders and all territories, with a Spanish version for Puerto Rico. What, if any, change in knowledge, attitudes or behaviour resulted from this massive and much-applauded effort? The brochure did elicit 250 000 calls to a special telephone hot-line. However, according to a Gallup Poll, 51% of a population sample queried said they had not read the report, either because they had no recollection of its arrival or because they chose not to read it when they saw it.[93] A national health interview survey undertaken in May and June 1988 revealed marginal gains in accurate information and marginal reductions in misinformation about AIDS in June as compared with May after mass distribution of the brochure.[94] Public funding for education projects must include a mandatory set-aside for evaluation of outcome,[88] lest we continue to invest in ineffective methods.

Although the prevalence of HIV infection among heterosexuals in the United States and Western Europe has remained relatively low, the 1 : 1 male/female ratio in Africa gives reason for concern that current rates may increase if preventive measures are not undertaken. Therefore, education about sexuality and STD transmission must be 'part of a comprehensive health education plan' in public schools, as stated by the Committee on School Health of the American Academy of Pediatrics.[95] The Committee recommends that concepts of health and disease, including the role of microorganisms, and the importance of cleanliness, should be the focus from kindergarten to third grade. From grades 4 to 6, the nature of AIDS and its modes of transmission should be included; myths of insect vectors and casual spread should be dispelled. Because risk behaviours are likely to begin at about grade 7, the Committee calls for an intensive secondary school curriculum with emphasis on AIDS as an STD, the nature of HIV infection and the immune response, modes of transmission (including intravenous drug use), the prevention and treatment of the disease, and discussion of its social and phychological aspects.

The Academy Committee has cautioned that: 'candid discussion of all aspects of sexual transmission must occur in an age-appropriate and culturally sensitive fashion.' The recommendations, while correct and straightforward in concept, are broad and general; their translation into specific educational content is the key to the success of the effort. Care will be required to avoid identifying sex so closely with disease as to impair normal sexual development. The literature on health education provides abundant evidence that presenting the facts is not enough.[96] Teenagers must be motivated to act and equipped with the skills to do so. A promising lead is provided by the success of classroom training programmes designed to augment behavioural skills in resisting the social pressure to conform with peer solicitations to begin smoking.[97,98]

Given the number of hours most citizens of the United States and Western European countries spend watching television, TV could become a highly effective way to reach the general population. Thus far, concern about offending the moral sensibility of some viewers has limited TV messages to general and non-specific presentations during other than prime time hours. Television networks, which have few reservations about soap operas which celebrate clandestine sex, demur at showing the ways sex can be made safer—for example, by displaying the proper way to use a condom. A state-supported TV campaign in the Dominican Republic has demonstrated that explicit programming about condom application lead to greater public knowledge and increased use.[99]

As emphasized from the beginning of this chapter, the problem of HIV infection transcends national boundaries. The epidemiology of AIDS differs between countries; control measures will have to take these differences into account; their effectiveness will depend on their sensitivity to unique features of culture and social matrix; the way ethical issues are resolved will differ by country but they are everywhere paramount. No country can isolate itself from the danger by instituting mandatory screening at its borders (as some have proposed doing). Effective actions require international cooperation.[100] The World Summit of Ministers of Health on Programmes for AIDS Prevention, meeting in London in January 1988,[101] declared that:

'The single most important component of national AIDS programmes is information and education because HIV transmission can be prevented through informed and responsible behaviour... [Such programmes] should take full account of social and cultural patterns, different lifestyles, and human and spiritual values ... We emphasize the need in AIDS prevention programmes to protect human rights and human dignity. Discrimination against, and stigmatization of, HIV infected people and people with AIDS and population groups undermine public health and must be avoided.'

In similar terms, the 41st World Health Assembly,[102] held in Geneva on 13 May 1988, resolved that member states be urged:

'To foster a spirit of understanding and compassion ... and to protect the human rights and dignity of HIV-infected people ... and to insure the confidentiality of HIV testing and to promote the availability of confidential counselling and other support services.'

REFERENCES

1. Mann, J.M. and Chin, J. AIDS, a global perspective. *N Engl J Med* 1988; **319**: 302–303.
2. Institute of Medicine. *Confronting AIDS: Update 1988*. Washington, D C: National Academy Press, 1988.

3. Centers for Disease Control. Pneumocystis pneumonia: Los Angeles. *Morb Mort Wkly Rep* 1981; **30**: 250–252.
4. Edman, J.C., Kovacs, J.A., Masur, H., Santi, D.V., Elwood, H.J. and Sogin, M.L. Ribosomal RNA sequence shows *Pneumocystis carinii* to be a member of the Fungi. *Nature* 1988; **344**: 519–522.
5. Centers for Disease Control. Kaposi's sarcoma and pneumonocystis pneumonia among homosexual men: New York City and California. *Morb Mort Wkly Rep* 1981; **30**: 305–308.
6. Ross, R.K., Casagrande, J.T., Dworsky, R.L., Levine, A. and Mack, T. Kaposi's sarcoma in Los Angeles, California. *J Natl Cancer Inst* 1985; **75**: 1011–1015.
7. Walzer, P.D., Perl, D.P., Krogstad, D.J., *et al*. *Pneumocystis carinii* pneumonia in the United States: epidemiologic diagnostic and clinical features. *Ann Intern Med* 1974; **80**: 83–98.
8. AIDS Program, Center for Infectious Disease, Centers for Disease Control. United States cases reported to CDC. *AIDS Weekly Surveillance Report*, November 28, 1988.
9. Friedman, S.R., Sotheran, J.L., Abdul-Quader, A., *et al*. The AIDS epidemic among blacks and Hispanics. *Milbank Mem Fund* 1987; **65**: Suppl. 2:455–499.
10. Allen, J.R. and Curran, J.W. Prevention of AIDS and HIV infection: needs and priorities for epidemiologic research. *Am J Publ Hlth* 1988; **78**: 381–386.
11. Barre-Sinoussi, F., Chermann, J.C., Rey, F., *et al*. Isolation of a T-lymphotropic retrovirus from a patient at risk for acquired immune deficiency syndrome (AIDS). *Science* 1983; **220**: 868–871.
12. Gallo, R.C., Sarin, P.S., Gelmann, E.P. *et al*. Isolation of human T-cell leukemia virus in acquired immune deficiency syndrome (AIDS). *Science* 1983; **220**: 865–867.
13. Duesberg, P. HIV is not the cause of AIDS. *Science* 1988; **241**: 514.
14. Blattner, W., Gallo, R.C. and Temin, H.M. HIV causes AIDS. *Science* 1988; **241**: 515–517.
15. Osborn, J.E. The AIDS epidemic: six years. *Ann Rev Pub Hlth* 1988; **9**: 551–583.
16. Fischl, M.A., Richman, D.D., Grieco, M.H., *et al*. The efficacy of azidothymidine (AZT) in the treatment of patients with AIDS and AIDS-related complex: a double-blind, placebo-controlled trial. *N Engl J Med* 1987; **317**: 185–191.
17. Dournon, E., Rozenbaum, W., Michon, C., *et al*. Effects of zidovudine in 365 consecutive patients with AIDS or AIDS-related complex. *Lancet* 1988; **ii**: 1297–1302.
18. DeWit, R., Boucher, C.A.B., Veenhof, K.H.N., *et al*. Clinical and virological effects of high-dose recombinant interferon-alpha in disseminated AIDS-related Kaposi's sarcoma. *Lancet* 1988; **ii**: 1214–1217.
19. Lane, H.C., Feinberg, J., Davey, V. *et al*. Anti-retroviral effects of interferon-alpha in AIDS-associated Kaposi's sarcoma. *Lancet* 1988; **ii**: 1218–1222.
20. Marx, J.L. The AIDS virus can take on many guises. *Science* 1988; **241**: 1039–1040.
21. Preston, B.D., Poiesz, B.J. and Loeb, L.A. Fidelity of HIV-I reverse transcriptase. *Science* 1988; **242**: 1168–1171.
22. Roberts, J.D., Bebenek, K. and Kunkel, T.A. The accuracy of reverse transcriptase from HIV-I. *Science* 1988; **242**: 1171–1173.
23. Koff, W.C. and Hoth, D.F. Development and testing of AIDS vaccines. *Science* 1988; **241**: 426–431.
24. Eisenberg, L. The genesis of fear: AIDS and the public's response to science. *Law, Med Hlth Care* 1986; **14**: 243–249.
25. Brandt, A.M. AIDS in historical perspective: four lessons from the history of sexually transmitted diseases. *Am J Publ Hlth* 1988; **78**: 367–371.
26. Curran, J.W., Lawrence, D.N., Jaffe, H., *et al*. AIDS associated with transfusions. *N Engl J Med* 1984; **310**: 69–75.

27. Evatt, B.L. Ramsley, R.B., Lawrence, D.N., Zylka, L.D. and Curran, J.W. AIDS in patients with hemophilia. *Ann Intern Med* 1984; **100**: 499–504.
28. Harris, C.A., Small, C.B., Klein, R.S., *et al*. Immunodeficiency in female sexual partners of men with AIDS. *N Engl J Med* 1983; **308**: 1181–1184.
29. Scott, G.B., Fischl, M.A., Klimas, N. *et al*. Mothers of infants with AIDS: evidence for both symptomatic and asymptomatic carriers. *J Am Med Assoc* 1985; **253**: 363–366.
30. Stenart, G.J., Tyler, J.P.P., Cunningham, A.L., *et al*. Transmission of HHTLV-III by artificial insemination by donor. *Lancet* 1985; **ii**: 581–584.
31. Centers for Disease Control. AIDS and HIV infection among health care workers. *Morb Mort Wkly Rep* 1988; **37**: 229–234.
32. Mulder, C. Human AIDS virus not from monkeys. *Nature* 1988; **333**: 396.
33. Smith, T.F., Srinivasan, A., Schochetman, G., Marcus, M. and Myers, G. The phylogenetic history of immunodeficiency viruses. *Nature* 1988; **333**: 573–575.
34. Curran, J.W., Jaffe, H.W., Hardy, A.M., Morgan, W.M. Selik, R.M. and Dondero, T.J. Epidemiology of HIV infection and AIDS in the United States. *Science* 1988; **239**: 610–616.
35. Piot, P., Plummer, F.A., Mhalu, F.S., Lamboray, J.-L., Chin, J. and Mann, J.M. AIDS: an international perspective. *Science* 1988; **239**: 573–579.
36. Simonsen, J.N., Cameron, W., Gakinya, M.N. *et al*. Human immunodeficiency virus infection among men with sexually transmitted disease. *N Engl J Med* 1988; **319**: 274–278.
37. Friedland, G.H. and Klein, R.S. Transmission of the human immunodeficiency virus. *N Engl J Med* 1987; **317**: 1125–1135.
38. Ward, J.W., Holmberg, S.D., Allen, J.R. *et al*. Transmission of HIV by blood transfusions screened as negative for HIV antibody. *N Engl J Med* 1988; **318**: 473–478.
39. Feldblum, P.J. and Fortney, J.A. Condoms, spermicides, and the transmission of human immunodeficiency virus. *Am J Publ Hlth* 1988; **78**: 52–54.
40. Fink, R. Changes in public reaction to a new epidemic: the case of AIDS. *Bull NY Acad Med* 1987; **63**: 939–949.
41. Dawson, D.A., Cynamon, M. and Fitti, J.E. AIDS knowledge and attitude for September 1987. NCHS Advance Data. Vital and Health Statistics of the National Center for Health Statistics. Number 148. 18 January 1988.
42. Landefeld, C.S., Chren, M.-M., Sega, J., Speroff, T. and McGuire, E. Students' sexual behavior, knowledge, and attitudes relating to the Acquired Immunodeficiency Syndrome. *J Gen Intern Med* 1988; **3**: 161–165.
43. Bass, A. Teen-agers seen ignoring AIDS advice. *Boston Globe* 14 August 1988, p. 8.
44. Moatti, J.P. Manesse, L., LeGales, C., Pages, J.P. and Fagnani, F. Social perception of AIDS in the general public: a French study. *Hlth Pol* 1988; **9**: 1–8.
45. Winkelstein, W., Samuel, M., Padian, N.S. *et al*. The San Francisco Men's Health Study. III: Reduction in HIV transmission among homosexual/bisexual men, 1982–1986. *Am J Publ Hlth* 1987; **77**: 685–689.
46. Martin, J.L. The impact of AIDS on gay male sexual pattens in New York City. *Am J Publ Hlth* 1987; **77**: 578–581.
47. FitzGerald, F. A reporter at large: The Castro-I. *The New Yorker*, pp. 34–70, 21 July 1986.
48. FitzGerald, F. The Castro-II. *The New Yorker*, pp. 44–63, 28 July 1986.
49. Centers for Disease Control. Syphilis and congenital syphilis—United States, 1985;1988. *Morb Mort Wkly Rep* 1988; **37**: 486–489.
50. Fineberg, H.V. Education to prevent AIDS: prospects and obstacles. *Science* 1988; **239**: 592–596.
51. Jones, E.F., Forrest, J.D., Goldman, N., *et al*. Teenage pregnancy in developed

countries: determinants and policy implications. *Fam Plan Perspect* 1985; **17**: 53–63.

52. Institute of Medicine/National Academy of Sciences. *Confronting AIDS: Directions for Public Health*. Washington DC: National Academy Press, 1986.
53. The Presidential Commission on the Human Immunodeficiency Virus Epidemic: *Report Submitted to the President of the United States*, 24 June 1988.
54. Richwald, G.A., Wamsley, M.A., Coulson, A.H. and Morisky, D.E. Are condom instructions readable? *Publ Hlth Rep* 1988; **103**: 355–359.
55. Sydenham, T. Cited in Temkin, O. Medicine and the problem or moral responsibility. *Bull Hist Med* 1949; **23**: 1–9.
56. Podhoretz, N. Cited in Dershowitz, A. Emphasize scientific information. *New York Times*, 19 March 1986.
57. Brandt, A.M. The syphilis epidemic and its relation to AIDS. *Science* 1988; **239**: 375–380.
58. Stokes, J.H. The practitioner and the antibiotic age of venereal disease control *J Ven Dis Inform* 1950; **31**: 1–13.
59. Tversky, A. and Kahneman, D. The framing of decisions and the psychology of choice. *Science* 1981; **211**: 453–458.
60. Fehrs, L.J., Foster, L.R., Fox, V., *et al*. Trial of anonymous versus confidential human immunodeficiency virus testing. *Lancet* 1988; **ii**: 379–382.
61. Ohi, G., Hasegawa, T., Kai, I. *et al*. Notification of HIV carriers: possible effect on uptake of AIDS testing. *Lancet* 1988; **ii**: 947–949.
62. Navia, B.A., Jordan, B.D. and Price, R.W. The AIDS dementia complex I. Clinical features. *Ann Neurol* 1986; **19**: 517–524.
63. Navia, B.A. and Price, R.W. The acquired immunodeficiency syndrome dementia complex as the presenting or sole manifestation of HIV infection. *Arch Neurol* 1987; **44**: 65–69.
64. Price, R.W., Brew, B., Sidtis, J., *et al*. The brain in AIDS: central nervous system HIV-1 infection and the AIDS dementia complex. *Science* 1988; **239**: 586–592.
65. Kessler, R.C., O'Brien, K., Joseph, J.G., *et al*. Effects of HIV infection, perceived health and clinical status on a cohort at risk for AIDS. *Soc Sci Med* 1988; **27**: 569–578.
66. Rose, R., Jenkins, C.D. and Hurst, M.W. *Air Traffic Controller Health Change Study*. Report to the Federal Aviation Administration. Boston, 1978 (privately published).
67. Skegg, D.C.G., Richards, S.M. and Doll, R. Minor tranquillizers and road accidents. *Br Med J* 1979; **i**: 917–919.
68. Graeber, R.C. Crew factors in flight operations: IV: Sleep and wakefulness in international aircrews. *NASA Technical Memorandum 88231*. NASA, 1986.
69. Torsvall, L. and Akerstedt, T. Sleepiness on the job: continuously measured EEG changes in train drivers. *Electroencephalogr Clin Neurophysiol* 1987; **66**: 502–511.
70. Institute of Medicine. *Airline Pilots: Age, Health and Performance*. Washington DC: National Academy Press, 1981.
71. Doege, T.C. Neurological and neurosurgical conditions associated with aviation safety. *Arch Neurol* 1979; **36**: 731–710.
72. Green, R. Aviation psychology. *Br Med J* 1983; **i**: 1880–1882.
73. Global Programme on AIDS: *Report of the Consultation on the Neuropsychiatric Aspects of HIV Infection*. Geneva: World Health Organization, March 14–17, 1988.
74. Cleary, P.D., Barry. M.J., Mayer, K.:H., Brandt, A.M., Gostin, L. and Fineberg, H.V. Compulsory premarital screening for the human immunodeficiency virus: technical and public health considerations. *J Am Med Assoc* 1987; **258**: 1757–1762.
75. Wilkerson, I. Illinoisans fault prenuptial AIDS tests. *New York Times*, 16 April 1988.

76. Associated Press. Required premarital AIDS test dealt 2 setbacks. *New York Times*, 29 April 1988.
77. Byrne, G. Crossing the border. Science 1988; **242**: 869.
78. Special Programme on AIDS. *Report of the Meeting on Criteria for HIV Screening Programmes*. Geneva: World Health Organisation, 20–21 May 1987.
79. Landesman, S., Minkoff, H., Holman, S., McCalla, S. and Sijin, O. Serosurvey of human immunodeficiency virus infection in parturients. *J Am Med Assoc* 1987; **258**: 2701–2703.
80. Hoff, R., Berardi, V.P., Weiblen, B.J., Mahoney-Trout, L. Mitchell, M.L. and Grady, G.F. Seroprevalence of human immunodeficiency virus among childbearing women. *N Engl J Med* 1988; **318**: 525–530.
81. Burke, D.S., Brundage, J.F., Redfield, R.R., *et al*. Measurement of false positive rate in a screening program for HIV infections. *N Engl J Med*. 1988; **319**: 961–964.
82. Mullis, K., Faloona, F., Scharf, S., Saiki, R., Horn, G. and Ehrlich, H. Specific amplification of DNA in vitro: the polymerase chain reaction. *Cold Spring Harbor Symp Quant Biol* 1986; **51**: 263–272.
83. Loche, M. and Mach, B. Identification of HIV-infected seronegative individuals by a direct diagnostic test based on hybridisation to amplified viral DNA. *Lancet* 1988; **ii**: 418–421.
84. Laure, F., Rouzioux, C., Verber, F., *et al*. Detection of HIV-1 DNA in infants and children by means of the polymerase chain reaction. *Lancet* 1988; **ii**: 538–541.
85. Weiss, R. and Tjhier, S. HIV testing is the answer—what's the question? *N Engl J Med* 1988; **319**: 1010–1012.
86. Cleary, P.D., Singer, E., Rogers, T.F., *et al*. Sociodemographic and behavioral characteristics of HIV antibody-positive donors. *Am J Publ Hlth* 1988; **78**: 953–957.
87. Cleary, P.D. Personal communication. September, 1988.
88. Chelimsky, E. Testimony before the Committee on Governmental Affairs, United States Senate, 8 June 1988. US General Accounting Office. GAO/T-PEMD-88-8.
89. Winkelstein, W., Wiley, J.S., Padian, N.S., *et al*. The San Francisco men's health study: continued decline in HIV seroconversion rates among homosexual/bisexual men. *Am J Publ Hlth* 1988; **78**: 1472–1474.
90. Parker, R. Acquired immunodeficiency syndrome in urban Brazil. *Med Anthropol Q* 1987; **1**: 155–175.
91. Stoneburner, R.L., Des Jarlais, D.C., Benezra, D., *et al*. A larger spectrum of severe HIV-I-related disease in intravenous drug users in New York City. *Science* 1988; **242**: 916–919.
92. Warwick, I., Aggleton, P. and Homans, H. Constructing commonsense—young people's beliefs about AIDS. *Sociol Health and Illness* 1988; **10**: 213–233.
93. Blendon, R.J. and Donelan, K. Discrimination against people with AIDS: the public's perspective. *N Engl J Med* 1988; **319**: 1022–1026.
94. Dawson, D.A. AIDS knowledge and attitudes for May and June 1988. NCHS Advance Data. *Vital and Health Statistics of the National Center for Health Statistics*. Number 160, 26 September 1988.
95. Committee on School Health, American Academy of Pediatrics: Acquired Immuno-deficiency Syndrome education in schools. *Pediatrics* 1988; **82**: 278–280.
96. Becker, M.H. and Joseph, J.G. AIDS and behavior change to reduce risk: a review. *Am J Publ Hlth*. 1988; **78**: 394–410.
97. Schinke, S.P., Gilchrist, L.D. and Snow, W.H. Skills intervention to prevent cigarette smoking among adolescents. *Am J Publ Hlth* 1985; **75**: 665–667.
98. Best, J.A., Thomson, S.J., Santi, S.M., Smith, E.A., Brown, K.S. Preventing cigarette smoking among school children. *Ann Rev Publ Hlth* 1988; **9**: 161–201.

99. Judy Foreman. Dominican Republic study. *Boston Globe*, January 1988.
100. Special Programme on AIDS. *Report of the Consultation on International Travel and HIV Infection*. Geneva: World Health Organization 2–3 March 1987.
101. World Summit of Ministers of Health. *London Declaration on AIDS Prevention*. 28 January 1988.
102. World Health Assembly. Avoidance of discrimination in relation to HIV infected people and people with AIDS. Resolution WHA 41.24, adopted 13 May 1988, Geneva.

CHAPTER 12

Ethics, Health Education, and Nutrition

POVL RIIS

SUMMARY

Lifestyles are very resistant to changes forced on the individual in both the subgroups of fundamental and of adopted lifestyles. This resistance is caused by cultural tradition and its geographical variation. Even within nations and local cultures the variation in eating and drinking habits is considerable. With this background it is obvious that health education represents a balance between ethnic and social tolerance on one side, and the need for active prevention on the other. The mere collection of scientific data on eating and drinking habits can include an ethically significant risk of stigmatizing certain groups. Health education can be applied *directly* or *indirectly*—the direct form deals with patients and the indirect with primary intervention in the shape of mass campaigns. Human nutrition is by nature complex and health education accordingly must be multifactorial. A special problem stems from health educators' moralistic bias which leads them— sometimes subconsciously—to adapt health education to their own life-habits in an attempt to avoid being targeted themselves, especially in sensitive matters such as alcohol consumption. A further problem is the impact on young people's eating and drinking habits rising from the behaviour of film and television heros. In this chapter I summarize a number of crucial questions in health education which can only be answered by reliable scientific information and not by guessing or finding smart slogans with public impact as their only value. Dealing with educational technique, I conclude that health education needs to be multidisciplinary to avoid amateurism in bringing scientific messages from its sources to the population.

FUNDAMENTAL AND ADOPTED LIFESTYLES

Lifestyles are as a whole very resistant to changes enforced upon the individual. This is true for adopted lifestyles such as alcohol consumption, dressing habits,

Ethics in Health Education
Edited by S. Doxiadis. ©1990 John Wiley & Sons Ltd

car driving practice, upbringing of children and so on, but it is even more true for fundamental lifestyles, crucial to survival and growth and induced very early in life, such as eating habits. Further resistance is represented by cultural tradition and its geographical variation which is nowadays even more widespread with the increasing numbers of multiethnic societies.

Because of the large number of refugees traversing the Earth's latitudes and longitudes, large groups of people now live under quite different climatic and cultural circumstances than those representing their country or culture of origin. Access to traditional food may then be difficult or impossible and the local food and amount of sunshine (linked to the production of, for instance, vitamin D) may all differ significantly from what was laid down by upbringing, education, and original tradition.

But even *within* nations and firm cultures subgroups might represent the combination of special life habits and inborn resistance to health education in eating and drinking habits. This is true, for example, for numbers of old and very old people, special lifestyle groups such as vegetarians and so on.

Thus, an overall ethical consideration is needed within this field of health education, with a balance between ethnic and social tolerance on one side, and the need for active prevention on the other. As in similar areas of medical epidemiology and clinical medicine, ethics are strongly linked to the practice of intervention, the age groups included, the scientific base, and the methods applied.

The mere collection of scientific data on eating and drinking habits might include an ethically significant risk of stigmatizing certain groups. But in most cases it is not the scientific knowledge in itself, but its projection to intervention programmes which raises the strongest ethical problems. Intervention can be an offer to be accepted or refused according to the citizen's free will, or it can be a forceful intervention decreasing the number of choices for the individual citizen, for instance by legally prescribing the addition of certain food additives to flour, milk, etc. It can even influence the way food is procured and processed. Orthodox Judaism, for example, prescribes certain methods of slaughtering, sometimes in conflict with national laws outlining methods of anaesthesia, physical techniques in slaughtering and so on.

DIRECT AND INDIRECT HEALTH EDUCATION

The health professions are to a large extent oriented towards *direct* health education as a part of their contact with patients. In case of a severe—or just avoided—health threat the citizen is maximally (yet not always optimally) motivated for secondary prevention. Further, the representative of the health profession and the professional knowledge is right there on the spot.

In this way nations consider health education to be in accordance with the usual expectations for, and norms of, the traditional patient–doctor relationship. This means that the information is considered reliable and directed towards the individual patient, not including societal aspects as cost for society in health care, pension, and so on. On the positive side of this patient–physician situation is the degree of motivation and mutual trust and reliability. On the negative side is the doctor's inclination not to stress health education further than is believed to be acceptable to the patient. Sometimes the truth would be more effective, but at the same time more shocking, than may seem appropriate in the pleasant atmosphere between patient and doctor.

Instead health administrators and health politicians rightly stress the importance of *indirect* health education, linked to primary intervention, and at the same time facing lesser motivation ('Why bother, it works well as it is') and a longer distance between health educator and citizens or target groups.

Here the problem is the large target groups not specifically motivated to listen to indirect health education. Among the reasons for this lack of motivation can be that they rightly want to live their own lives, and that they consider the choice of different life-habits as part of their personal responsibility and quality of life. Other reasons can include the difficulty in reaching such target groups by pamphlets, posters, newspaper campaigns etc. Possibly the electronic media represent the best access to such groups, but these channels are expensive and demanding and require specialized communication skills and techniques. One risk of applying modern advertisement techniques in the electronic media, when influencing eating and drinking habits, is an overpopularization of the serious topics, in this way often losing impact, when the simple strong signals subside in weeks or months.

These two levels of health education consequently create the dilemma—much needed, less obtainable—less needed, more obtainable. Dealing with nutrition and drinking habits this dilemma is obvious.

THE COMPLEX HEALTH INFLUENCES IN EATING AND DRINKING HABITS

Human nutrition is by nature complex, comprising a large number of quantitative and qualitative components, from trace elements and vitamins to essential amino-acids, dietary lipids, and total amount of calories. This means that health education within this area easily comes to share health targets (survival, rates for cancer, and for the ischaemic syndrome in all its appearances etc.) with other important long-ranging factors: genetics, smoking, occupational hazards, drug consumption. This oligo-target multi-factor problem creates another ethical and educational dilemma. To be influential health education will have to point to goals in citizens' lifetimes, and optimally will have to make the gains visible, not only in an anonymous statistical way, but preferably in a direct person-identifiable way. But to be scientifically valid and honest, the factual content of health educational schemes will have to be presented as what they are: complex and strongly varying when one goes from epidemiological figures to individual prognoses.

This procedure, to project group results to individuals represents probably one of the biggest educational challenges both inside the medical profession and from the profession to society. Many doctors dealing with clinical decision-making based on scientific evidence from controlled trials still have problems in applying such results to individual patients. Patients might even exploit the fact that their special case is not to the full extent comprised by the variation represented in an important controlled trial. To be open and fair in weighing such evidence in individual patient-doctor relationships means, unfortunately, a reduction of the authority of the doctor (a reduction however, regained in an increased credibility). In other words, patients who prefer a short perspective, and wish to preserve their free will, even in continuing unhealthy eating and drinking habits, will be able to find escape routes when society and its health representatives try to emphasize the longer perspectives of health and the importance of applying such perspectives by changing daily eating and drinking habits.

COUNTERBALANCING THE HEALTH EDUCATORS' MORALISTIC BIAS

Dealing with fundamental lifestyles such as nutrition, and a widespread adopted lifestyle such as alcohol usage, presents yet another difficulty in the short-term and long-term credibility of largescale health education. Problems of overweight and poorly controlled drinking will be a personal or close experience of many health workers and health education planners, whether met as a personal problem to be fought, or as a demonstrated fact among relatives or friends. The acknowledgment of such personal or close experiences are often regarded almost as taboo in modern societies. The fact that doctors, for example have, according to some statistics, an alcohol consumption approximately three times that of a background population means that the doctor and the patient often do *not* meet each other on a kind of mutual platform, enabling the doctor to be the professional advocate of the patient from a base of sympathy and technical or clinical knowlege.[1]

Many health professionals have not been able to counterbalance this personal bias. They either react with strong condemnation of obesity or alcohol addiction as 'sinful', self-inflicted diseases which are totally the responsibility of the patient, or they become resigned to their personal problem, thereby diminishing their credibility from the very beginning. The very obese, doctor instructing the newly diagnosed diabetic in the importance of calory control, for example, will not carry much authority, just as the words of the smoking thoracic surgeon will have little credibility for the emphysematic chronic smoker.

This mutual loss of credibility is often not recognized by the two individuals in the patient-doctor relationship. The doctor will try to persuade himself or herself that the patient does not know of or has not registered any personal eating or drinking problems of the doctor. On the other side, the patient might have the same confidence in his or her capability to disguise signs of food or alcohol addiction. Sometimes the number of plausible excuses and explanations in the patient's vocabulary seems to be inexhaustible.

To be able to compensate for such personal bias is an essential condition for all health educators. It is not the same as considering all lifestyles equal and thus losing an important educational dimension. As a whole no doctor or other health worker will be able to deal with important aspects of patients' or citizens' lives such as death, personal crises, eating and drinking habits, and so on, without having analysed *their own* attitudes and habits to the extent of painfully facing the true facts. A generation or two ago clinicians were taught to behave as neutrally as possible in dealing with the patients. This general rule implied, that doctors and other health personnel should not in any way disclose their personal life experience, their losses, their habits in eating and drinking and so on. The ideal was the neutral health system representative who only very indirectly disclosed her or his personal norms etc. in the way they dealt with the patient as a fellow human being. Nowadays the habits of doctors and other health workers have changed. Far from having ended in the opposite ditch, making for instance every patient-doctor meeting an exchange of very personal and existential statements, doctors and other health workers today include information on personal norms and habits, by sometimes reporting, and always removing, suspected personal bias from their advice on health education. In this way health professionals are exposed to a higher degree than earlier, but at the same time they have gained much more in reliability and confidence.

THE ANONYMOUS LIVES AND THE LIFESTYLES OF THE IDOLS

The life of modern man even in developing countries is to a large extent influenced by fiction, primarily in television, but also to a large extent in films. Dealing with the human body, its anatomy, physiology and clinical ways of reaction, the worldwide fiction industry again and again demonstrates its lack of knowledge, or even worse its cynical disregard for knowledge in presenting man as a biological creature. Think for instance of the large number of knockouts shown in films and video productions where the hero, after a blow to his jaw or head that would send anyone else into a long coma or even to a department of neurosurgery, jumps to his feet after a few seconds, shakes his head, and resumes all his vigorous actions, as expected from the hero species. The severe brain concussion, the epidural or subdural haemorrhage, and other possible consequences appear to be non-existent.

The same seductive lack of realism can be seen in the way the strong influence of alcohol can suddenly subside when the hero needs all his or her capabilities to be a hero in the next sequences of the film or video. Here again there is no disturbing or inconvenient fact of alcohol metabolism and the physiologically determined time factor, only the director's and producer's need for fast action and continuation of the plot.

Alcohol is particularly in focus as a part of human eating and drinking habits depicted again and again in films and video productions. It is often used as a macho symbol, intending to show that the capability of drinking a great deal of alcohol and still being able to function is a special sign of strength and maturity, especially in men. The truth is, of course, that these kind of norms are more linked to men's post-pubertal boasting to disguise their insecurity, than to the grown-up responsible male, whether in real life or in the fictional character. For the experienced spectator such a false picture of human maturity will do very little but create a weary scepticism. But for the sensitive young person the link between strength, importance, and mastery of the situation and alcohol consumption (or smoking) might have very negative consequences in creating a kind of Pavlovian reflex between the much wanted central role in a group and the habit of excessive alcohol drinking. Similarly, the film and video scenes where people in crises or suddenly captured stretch their hand out for a drink almost as a reflex action can be a potent influence on the impressionable. In this way fiction adds to the illusion that any mental shock or suprise is best remedied by alcohol consumption and not by spontanous emotion combined with thought.

Another stereotypic role of alcohol consumption in films and video productions is that of mad driving after alcohol consumption. This only depicts the picturesque in a row of near-disasters which never happen (unless the driver is one of the villains). Again we do not see the fractures, the cerebral haemorrhages, the misery, the innocent victims hit and killed and so on.

Eating habits are also influenced by fiction. Meals in the film industry only serve pleasure, often to the extent of gluttony. A special, and refined, use of eating is meals as a symbolic sexual activity. Favourite actors and especially actresses have a strong influence on the eating habits of older children's and young people's choice of their ideal body weight and image. When actresses idolized by millions of teenagers are of the very skinny hunting dog type, such a model pushes young girls towards the anorexia end of the scale of human body weight variation. This is not to say that such fiction is *the* reason for an increase in numbers of cases of anorexia nervosa, but undoubtedly the influence of such heroes overwhelms much of the advice given by doctors, parents, or teachers.

RELIABLE SCIENTIFIC INFORMATION AS A NECESSARY BASE FOR HEALTH EDUCATION

The need for reliable information in health education represents a place where ethics and science meet prevention. Many health education schemes have been too ambitious in stretching the underlying scientific evidence to the breaking point, especially in the long run. In eating and drinking habits the need for better answers to basic questions *before* major educational programmes can be implemented is obvious. Many examples are at hand.

When doctors, other health personnel, and even whole institutions deal with human obesity, it has since long been considered simply the result of habitual overeating. But is this really true? Are the mechanisms behind overweight that simple? And, consequently, can this weight variation be dealt with by clinicians as just a problem of eating more than the person needs? The truth is, that we still know all too little about different subgroups of human obesity, probably only linked together by the simple message given by the weighing scale. It is also true that our measures of human metabolism expressed by oxygen consumption are probably all too crude to understand the mechanisms behind obesity. Research results seem to indicate that obese people do not eat more than slim people and that other mechanisms exist, removing the clinical entity, obesity, from a postulated group of self-inflected diseases involving an insufficient amount of self-control. Further, we know too little about possible genetic factors, influencing the control of hunger and satisfaction in man. New research results enable us to understand human obesity much better. They will provide a much more solid base for health education in eating habits, and thus will help to improve such education's ethical standards.[2,3]

At the opposite end of the body weight variation scale from obesity lies anorexia. Again we know all too little about the complex mechanisms leading to this sometimes life-threatening type of emaciation. Are genetic factors involved? Can we allow ourselves to consider anorexia simply as a deviation of psychological mechanisms from those involved in normal weight people? As in human obesity, have we not based health education and even campaigns on insufficient scientific evidence? Do we understand the complex psychological and physiological processes comprising satisfaction sufficiently to embark in mass campaigns for the prevention of anorexia? Is it sufficiently elucidated that non-eating is a kind of weapon for the young girl finding herself in strong interfamily conflicts? Or will we have to consider anorexia as a coarse headline diagnosis which includes subgroups of disease entities with different underlying mechanisms, just as has been the case in human obesity?[4,5]

In the industrialized countries overconsumption, and lack of physical exercise, have created a need for technical matters to avoid ischaemic diseases of the heart, brain, peripheral arteries and so on. The low prevalence of such diseases in the Inuit (Greenland Eskimoes) has led to the important observation that the reason for this low prevalence might be the high ingestion of N-3 polyunsaturated fatty acids in the arctic and subarctic regions. This has further led to the hope, that individuals of different ethnic groups who do not live in arctic areas might gain the same low prevalence of ischaemic diseases by a much higher ingestion of N-3 polyunsaturated fatty acids in their daily life. A number of important research results have demonstrated the influence of such polyunsaturated fatty acids on cellular processes, growth of neoplasms, coagulation processes etc.[6] In this way much support has been gathered for the idea of a beneficial effect of food supplements of N-3 polyunsaturated fatty acids. However the ultimate scientific proof of a beneficial influence on disease prevalences and especially survival is still lacking. Large-scale controlled trials, comparing intervention and control groups in a randomized double-blind way, have not given the necessary clear-cut answers. Despite the lack of scientific confirmation, the vacuum of reliable knowledge has already been invaded by commercial firms by making food supplements of N-3 polyunsaturated fatty acids popular sales items. However, to act in an ethically acceptable way, health administrators and planners will need more scientific results before large-scale campaigns on the desirability of widespread ingestion of these fatty acids can be defended.

Another much debated aspect of human health education in eating habits is the importance of a high fibre content and its possible influence on the risk of gastroenterological cancer in man. Can one turn the observation that populations with a low risk of such cancers have a high fibre consumption to a beneficial effect on cancer prevalences in other societies with low fibre consumption, if fibre is added to the food?[7] Do we possess enough evidence at present to justify large-scale nutritional health campaigns?

And what about salt (sodium chloride)? Will the amount of salt ingested influence the blood pressure level in non-hypertensive citizens? Our part of the world has seen large campaigns against salt, mainly run by industry. In this way this very basic constituent of our bodies has been invested almost with the status of a poison. And yet we do not know for sure if the fact that hypertensive patients must avoid a high salt consumption, in order not to increase their blood pressure, can be converted to a statement that non-hypertensive citizens will have to avoid a high salt consumption in order to stay normotensive. The resources involved in such campaigns, which almost create dual types of many kinds of food—for instance, normal salt/low salt—are formidable. Again industry seems to have filled the vacuum in the absence of reliable scientific information.

Trace elements, such as selenium, represent one of the latest waves of almost religious belief in remedies that might prevent people from getting cancer.[7] We seem to know too little of what is considered a safe consumption of selenium in our part of the world, and we know too little about the actual preventive benefit obtained by adding selenium to peoples' daily food. Again, the threat of severe diseases such as cancer (or ischaemic heart disease or brain diseases) facilitates private and commercial campaigns long before we possess an ethically acceptable level of information.

A main component in unhealthy drinking habits is alcohol. Again we need much more scientific evidence before being able to plan effective public campaigns on the health risks of overconsumption. Is consumption and overconsumption of alcohol simply a matter of personal choice or are genetic factors involved, implying in this way a risk of becoming an alcoholic in certain families?[8] In dealing with the public and with individual patients we still do not know enough about the safe limits for daily consumption of alcohol in women and men. Instead of trying to condemn alcohol as such (which has been very unsuccessful in all historical examples), we ought to be able to teach people to live with alcohol in a safe way, if they choose not to be totally abstinent as a part of their personal lifestyle. Instead of prescribing the doctors' personal consumption as constituting safe limits, it would be much better to have safe figures for the amounts not leading to increased figures for diseases and accidents. In this way we might even be able to plan the health education of children and young people in order to avoid early addiction to alcohol.

Even in treating alcoholics, we need more scientific evidence about the effect of so-called safe drinking as a reliable strategy. Instead of aiming at total abstinence for the rest of such patients' lifetimes, possibly supported by disulfiram, there would be great advantages if new and much more modest drinking habits could help at least larger subgroups of former alcohol addicts.

Central to the prevention of alcohol addition is much better knowledge of the ages at which alcohol habits are founded psychologically. Do such habits start much earlier than we believe? Do they reflect family members and other grown-ups' way of living, watched by the small child, long before it knows the concepts of alcohol consumption, addiction and so on?

To wait for more reliable scientific information on those topics, and many others, could lead to a kind of defeatism in which any initiative could be postponed because 'we still do not know enough.' Such a paralysis of intervention is not what is needed and nor is hasty, intervention schemes not based on satisfactory evaluation. The ideal is to transform reliable research results into active intervention through health education in a constantly progressive way. This implies that scientific development sets the pace in the long run, and that we indirectly determine this pace by supporting research within these important areas.

HEALTH EDUCATION NEEDS TO BE MULTIDISCIPLINARY

Based on the concept that amateurism (or its euphemism 'non-professionalism') constitutes a serious, sometimes even unethical, drawback in health education, such an endeavour implies a number of disciplines, that are by nature *not* health disciplines. Educational techniques are one such discipline. Health professionals are not normally trained and skilled in teaching, and such insights are of paramount importance. In the huge cacophony of modern advertising it needs skill to get a serious, clear-cut signal through to people, especially because reliable information has more inborn nuances, and—as all expressions of truth—moves rather slowly.

Sociology is another supportive discipline. A thorough knowledge of the norms, habits, traditions, and social forces in different age groups and social strata is seriously needed in planning campaigns for healthier eating and drinking habits.

Psychology too is another essential discipline. Reaching the target groups without creating adverse reactions presupposes familiarity with psychological reactions and the all-important concept, *retention*.

CONCLUSION

Where do we stand today in planning health education that is ethically acceptable within the field of nutrition and drinking habits? We face problems that range globally from the basic question of having enough food in one area to the prevention of overeating and indulgence in another, and that further range from cultures where religion makes alcoholism a small or non-existent problem to cultures where alcohol is arguably the major problem. Strategies for international organizations must of course vary accordingly.

Those who belong to the medical profession still often confuse personal experience (and even prejudices) with health education in a biased, moralistic way. To help the profession to be aware of this interaction is still a major task on the internal front. We lack scientific answers to a large number of fundamental questions dealing with food and drink. This fact should not paralyse us but should encourage us to concentrate our forces on those areas where our insight is greatest and reliable. We also lack a tradition for making health education multidisciplinary through cooperation among disciplines of identical scientific standards, instead of referring such cases to advertisement agencies.

We need to move on from here with stronger efforts in promoting indirect, primary health education. The eating and drinking habits of young people in the Western World is just one example of such urgently needed initiatives.

REFERENCES

1. Plant, M.A. Risk factors in employment. In Hore, B.D, Plant, M.A. (eds.). *Alcohol problems in employment*. London: Croom Helm, 1981.
2. Vague, J, Björntorp, P., Guy-Grand, O. *et al*. *Metabolic Complications of Human Obesities*. Amsterdam: Excerpta Medica, 1985.
3. Hey, H., Pedersen, H.D., Andersen, T., and Quaade, F. Formula diet with a free additional food choice up to 1000 kcal (4.2 MJ) compared with isoenergetic conventional diet in the treatment of obesity: a randomized clinical trial. *Ugeskr Laeger* 1986; **148**: 2741–2744.
4. Tolstrup, K. Anorexia nervosa. In Vejlsgaard, R. (ed.). *Medicinsk Arbog*. Copenhagen: Munksgaard, 1981.
5. Theander, S. Anorexia nervosa: a psychiatric investigation of 94 female patients. *Acta Psychiatr Scand* 1974; suppl. 214.
6. Fifth Acta Medica Scandinavica Symposium: No.3. Fatty Acids in Health and disease. Tromsö, Norway, August 11–13 1989.
7. Danish Society of Gastroenterology. Colorectal cancer—is prevention possible. Herlev University Hospital, February 10–11, 1989.
8. Conn, HO. Cirrhosis: genetic disposition to cirrhosis. In Schiff, L. (ed.). *Diseases of the Liver*. 4th edition. Philadelphia, Toronto: Lippincott, 1975.

CHAPTER 13

Health Education and Mental Health

JACQUELINE M. ATKINSON

SUMMARY

Education for positive mental health is beset by practical and ethical issues. This seems to have lead to a concentration of effort on areas of behaviour which are generally agreed to be problems or illnesses. For a variety of reasons the promotion of positive mental health does not seem to be valued in the same way as the promotion of positive physical health. This reflects difficulties in defining the concept of mental health, uncertainties in how best to achieve mental health, and resistance from political, social, and economic powers to overturn aspects of the system which contribute to mental distress.

INTRODUCTION

Mental health is a much neglected area of health education. The *Health Education Journal*, produced by the Health Education Authority is widely read by practitioners in the field in Britain. Over the past five years (1984–1988) its coverage of mental health has been minimal, with only five articles directly targeted at mental health. One was a general article on 'men, women and mental health',[1] one was on 'menstrual blues',[2] one on anxiety management,[3] one on community mental health,[4] and one on relationships in the mentally handicapped.[5] Related issues of alcohol and drug and substance abuse accounted for a further 19 articles. This must be set against a wide coverage of topics such as smoking and AIDS. Indeed, there have been 33 articles on AIDS including one whole issue in 1987. Yet the prevalence of mental illness and distress is considerably greater than that of AIDS. Why is mental health second class in health education? Are the reasons practical, or do they have an ethical basis? Do the two overlap? Is it because we do not really know what good mental health is? Or is it because of the approaches which would have to be taken?

Ethics in Health Education
Edited by S. Doxiadis. ©1990 John Wiley & Sons Ltd

Concepts of mental health are numerous, but definitions tend to describe *ill-health* rather than a more positive *well-being*, which is often labelled as the absence of 'illness'. Such definitions indicate that a medical model predominates in our thinking. What implications does that have for mental health education? Very few researchers have even begun to tackle this issue.[6]

It has been argued that Cartesian dualism 'has greatly enhanced biomedical technology by liberating the study of man from medieval theology. Legitimizing the study of the human body as a thing, that is, as a physical entity...has made possible great technical advances that could not have occurred if anatomical dissections and other experiments that might have challenged the authority of the church were prohibited.'[7] The legacy of the Cartesian approach may have freed much of medicine but it has left some problems for medical ethics, psychiatry, and health education. These disciplines usually want to view the person as a whole, an integrated being of body and mind living in an historical and cultural environment. This sits uneasily with the Cartesian split, which leads medicine to formulate problems as *either* mentalistic *or* materialistic.

WHAT IS MENTAL HEALTH?

There is broad agreement both within and between cultures about many aspects of physical health: a healthy, functioning heart is a healthy functioning heart whichever culture it beats in. Can the same be said of a healthy mind? A mind that functions well within the society in which it lives might be the only common ground. There may be broad agreement both within and between cultures about what constitutes major mental illness, but the attributes of positive mental health are more elusive. 'Normal' behaviour and 'normal' personality are related to mental health, more than physical attributes are related to physical health. A person's physical attractiveness is not automatically assumed to correlate with their physical health. A personality which is outside the 'average' is, however, likely to be associated with views of that person's mental health. Indeed there are psychiatric categories of 'personality disorder' which seems to suggest that this is an acceptable stance to take.

Some areas of body and mind are accepted as linked in many cultures, but not always meaning the same thing. Weight loss is accepted as common in depression in the Western diagnosis, and other cultures concur with this, such as the Havik[8] and Tunisians.[9] The difference comes with attitudes to plumpness. In Western society it is generally regarded that there is something 'wrong' with the person (most often women) and that what is 'wrong' is psychological.[10] Both the Havik and Tunisians however, associate reasonable weight gain with emotional well-being and a 'worry-free' attitude.

Since the range of personality types varies between cultures, so will the perception of 'normal' mental health. Extraversion and introversion, as measured by the EPI vary between cultures.[11] Problems become associated with less valued personalities, so that shyness, at least in popular descriptions of introversion, becomes associated with that personality type. Introversion is, of course, not to do with being shy but a particular way of relating to novelty in the environment.

Responses to behaviour, and its impact on society, will alter in accord with changes in the environment or culture. Thus, during time of war the special attributes of the psychopathic personality may make him peculiarly successful, only to find such attributes devalued, not to say opposed, in time of peace.

The definition of 'normal' personality or behaviour depends then on the perceptions of the observer and the relationship of the behaviour to the culture in which it is being performed. Although there is confusion between what is 'normal' and what is 'average', the two terms are often used interchangeably. The bounds of 'normal' might be stretched slightly beyond the two standard deviations on the normal distribution curve, but shades of grey eventually become black and an individual's personality or behaviour becomes labelled 'odd'. What one person labels as 'peculiarly odd' may be described by another as 'charmingly eccentric'. The description of behaviour is influenced by the describer's closeness to it. Thus we may be motivated to judge our own behaviour as normal but the same behaviour in another may bring forth censure. This leads to some extremely irregular verbs:

> I'm sensitive
> You're highly strung
> She's neurotic

Inevitably then, educating for positive mental health means that value judgments will be made. Downie and Fyfe in their consideration of health education in schools (Chapter 9) explain why there is 'no other subject on the curriculum which is so value-driven'. And no part of health education is more value-driven than mental health, and thus it cannot escape ethical consideration. Changing fashions and trends prescribe attitudes and behaviours, usually purporting to be the 'real' essence of Man.

The 1960s and 1970s saw an upsurge in psychological theories devoted to the development of the self. Theorists and therapists such as Erich Fromm, Carl Rogers, Abraham Maslow, Rollo May, Eric Berne, and Fritz Perls among others presented visions of positive mental health and ways to achieve it through their theories or brand of psychotherapy. Phrases summing up their philosophy passed into the language: 'I'm O.K.—You're O.K.' Everybody 'heard' but few listened. One of the cornerstones of many of these psychotherapies was openness, both in freedom to express feelings and to discover and explore sex. Promiscuity was outlawed as a concept, open marriages were promoted,[12] and guides for what was called 'recreational sex' abounded, ranging from the enormously popular *Joy of Sex*[13] to esoteric guides such as *Beginner's Guide to Group Sex*.[14]

As we move into the 1990s these views stand challenged, and not only because of the emergence of AIDS. There will always be divisions between those who see sexual freedom (usually taken to include a value-laden number of partners) as a sign of psychological health, and anything less as repression, and those who see 'excess' freedom as promiscuity and a sign of immaturity or an inability to form lasting relationships. Who is to say which embodies the greater truth? Which allows free reign to the true nature of Man? Or Woman? Our attitudes to sexual behaviour stem from deeply rooted moral beliefs and thus sex education is probably more controversial than any other area of health education. It is not possible to teach, or discuss sex education from anything other than an ethical basis.

Leaving this for less controversial issues we can return to the expression of emotion. Advocated by the self-promoting psychologies the expression of emotion became a central goal of positive mental health and personal growth. Ideas and practices arising mainly on the West Coast of the United States of America, a highly individual culture in its own right, were transplanted across the world, usually travelling less well than Californian wine.

A superficial examination of cultures shows, however, that the expression of emotions and other social behaviour varies widely, and the healthy in one culture will be defined as unhealthy in another. Northern European reserve and 'stiff-upper-lip' could be interpreted as 'withdrawal' or even 'lack of appropriate affect' in another culture. Afro-Caribbean culture expects a stronger expression of emotions, has a 'love of word-play and teasing use of language'[15] and often deeply held religious beliefs expressed in direct personal terms, which to Northern European perceptions can be labelled thought disorder. This misperception of cultural differences has led to controversy over the diagnosis of many people of Afro-Caribbean origins as suffering from schizophrenia.[16,17]

Because definitions of mental health tend not to go beyond the absence of distress we are left with a wide variety of styles of psychosocial functioning which seem to correlate with good mental health. The consequences of one lifestyle compared to another may affect health both directly and indirectly. Western culture is broadly competitive, although there are groups which would advocate cooperation. It is impossible to say which is more 'natural'. The consequences of either can be both positive or negative. Being competitive can produce rewards if the individual 'wins', both materially and psychologically (a sense of achievement, success, excitement, challenge) but can also encourage suspiciousness, lack of closeness, selfishness as well as stress, and feelings of pressure. A sense of well-being and closeness achieved through cooperation can be offset by a lack of material rewards in a system geared to competition, with subsequent bitterness or resentment. This is further complicated by health (both physical and mental) having a positive correlation with material rewards as measured by social class. Having the money to live in a middle class area gives the individual access to resources both directly and indirectly linked to health that are denied those living in areas of social deprivation.

It is interesting that even in the home of the competitive lifestyle, the United States, where 'nice guys finish last', a character such as Eddie 'the Eagle' Edwards should have found such national popularity (via Johnny Carson as well as the Olympics) encompassing as he does such concepts as 'amateurism' and 'playing the game' rather than winning. Could this possibly suggest that being 'a nice guy' is sometimes better than winning?

Albert Ellis's[18] approach to mental health and psychological distress moves towards combining rationality with emotion. Ellis believes that emotions come from the things the individual says to her or himself and negative emotions are based in irrational beliefs and the habit of catastrophizing. Although most people can accept the belief 'I must be liked by everyone' is irrational if carried to extremes and can only lead to insecurity, anxiety, depression, and other negative outcomes, they may find accepting the suggestion that we should not judge people on a 'good-bad' scale harder. This contradicts some religious, philosophical, or psychological assessments of human nature as fundamentally evil, violent, sinning, or otherwise negative.

Religions have usually advocated ways of living as well as particular beliefs, and many psychotherapies stand opposed to such strictures. The teachings of Thomas à Kempis[19] may strike many as overly restrictive: 'Open not thy heart to every man, but discuss thy business with one that is wise and feareth God. Be rarely with young people and strangers.' We recognize them, however, as teachings within a strict ethical code and system of belief to clearly defined ends: 'He that followeth Me walketh not in darkness, saith the Lord.'

Psychotherapy, or even education, rarely sets out its endpoint so clearly. It has been argued[20] that 'psychology has become a religion, in particular a form of secular humanism based on worship of the self.' Although many stand opposed to the strictures of religious teaching because of its damaging impact on mental health, rarely is the possible negative impact of psychology considered. Vitz, however, argues that 'Psychology as a religion has for years been destroying individuals, families and communities.'[20]

That religions or philosophies have a contribution to make to positive mental health and education is accepted. Thus a book taking a Christian approach to stress management[21] or anxiety[22] does not seem out of place, whereas 'A Christian approach to weight loss' or 'A Jewish guide to not smoking' would seem distinctly odd.

Although psychotherapies claim to be, if not always value-neutral, then at least non-judgmental, this is not always the case. Character, when considered by psychoanalysts, is concerned with the development of morality, and is thus not value- or culture-free. Freud went so far as to comment:

'If the physician has to deal with a worthless character, he soon loses the interest which makes it possible for him to enter profoundly into the patient's mental life. Deep rooted malformations of character, traits of an actually degenerate constitution, show themselves during treatment as sources of a resistance that can scarcely be overcome.'[23]

For some people, then, there would seem to be little hope.

Thus the foremost ethical dilemma the health educationalist faces is to decide what mental health is, and what aspects to promote. Coupled with this must be concern that by promoting certain attitudes, behaviours, or even personalities as 'more healthy' this might be seen as limiting the range of what *is* 'normal'. If a particular personality of behavioural attribute is *only* less successful because other people do not like it, the two approaches could be to change the behaviour, or teach others to be more tolerant. The former limits the boundaries of human variety, with all the attendant dangers that labelling others 'different' brings. I will return to this later in the chapter. The second approach assumes that heterogeneous socities are 'better' than homogeneous. Is this true?

Before either of these approaches can be evaluated however, there is a need to understand the causes of mental distress or mental ill health. This is not the place to try to answer these questions, but central issues such as whether the problem is located in the individual or society must be faced. The possible genetic component of some mental illnesses raises yet other ethical issues including those implicit in genetic counselling. Most psychotherapies locate the problem within the individual, ranging through unhealthy functioning of a dynamic unconscious to faulty learning experiences. Against this must be set the extensive evidence that psychological distress (and some mental illness) is positively correlated with adverse social conditions.[24] Establishing causal links is, however, beset with methodological problems.

Thus political, social, economic, and moral judgments are made if health education (or any other approach to psychological distress) accepts that it must not make social problems appear as problems of the person by individualizing therapy or education and thus supporting an inequitable system.

EDUCATION FOR POSITIVE MENTAL HEALTH

There are, therefore, two major approaches to promoting mental health: the micro approach, of altering an individual's behaviour and the macro, or political approach of reducing social inequalities. These two approaches reflect general concerns in health education as to outcomes for individuals, groups or the whole population. The option of changing society's view of people with problems will be dealt with later since it reflects more on mental illness than mental health.

Many of the social factors correlated with poor mental health are the same as those linked with poor physical health. The practical approaches to changing the socioeconomic antecedents has been discussed in detail elsewhere.[24] Ethical considerations range from whether all 'deserve' access to the same resources to how the change might be brought about (revolution or education).

Is aiming mental health education at individuals any easier? Is there agreement about how it might be done? Exposure to American culture via the media, where Woody Allen has done more than Freud to popularize psychotherapy, may lead to an assumption that some form of professional help or guidance is necessary. As more resources are targeted at helping individuals in physical health education to lose weight, take up exercise, or stop smoking but few expect to plumb the depths (or even the shallows) of their psyche without a therapist/lifeguard to assist them.

A recent review[25] in the United States has counted more than 400 different psychotherapies. Despite current trends towards eclecticism the unwary is still left with a bewildering choice. Eclecticism, as defined by Beitman and colleagues[26] is the use of procedures from various sources without, most importantly, necessarily accepting the underlying theories. Although this might be a worrying trend to many, viewing eclecticism as a 'worn out synonym for theoretical laziness' is rejected by the authors.

Rather than concentrating on intrapsychic events, another approach is to look at individual lifestyle. Does research given any indication of particular events and behaviours which contribute to psychological distress or poor mental health? It is worth noting that although considerable research effort is expended on the antecedents of 'problems' there is very little research on the causes of positive psychological states. To explore the reasons for this in detail is largely outwith the scope of this chapter, but must include sources of research funding and a general lack of interest in positive emotions or psychological states. It is well known that when psychologists research or report on topics such as 'love' or 'happiness' the popular press usually derides their efforts, states that what is found is 'common sense' and generally wonders why anyone might be interested. Is this because there is a fear that by 'tampering with' positive emotions we might somehow loose them? Do we want 'love' and 'happiness' to retain some element of magic and mystery? Even Ellis in his book on rational-emotive therapy[18] suggests leaving positive emotions alone and not examining them. Is the philosophy 'if it's not broken don't mend it'? Where does that leave fine tuning? Examining the causes of distress, however, gives us an opportunity to mend what has started to break; staying with the cliche philosophy 'a stitch in time...'

The area where health education has put most of its effort, in part at government insistence, has been alcohol, drug, and substance abuse. Why should this be? Is it, at least in part, because by stressing an individual health education approach political and ethical philosophies emphasizing personal responsibility are strengthened, blame is put on the individual for being 'weak', and the role of political and social forces in the development of such problems can more easily be ignored. Although drug and substance abuse can be devastating both psychologically and physically for the individual concerned they are nevertheless problems for only a small percentage of the population. Alcohol presents problems for many more. All are popular media topics, encompassing 'human interest' stories of tragedy, scandal, or pathos, or political exposes of corrupt business. The insidious problems presented, particularly by the use of alcohol, can however, on occasions, give rise to the media introducing its own health education and behaviour change campaigns.[27] Although there is general agreement about the preventative aspects of warnings against abuse of alcohol, drugs, and other substances, it is recognized that once again health education is giving a negative message. 'Don't do this' and prevent problems. Are there any 'do this' and prevent problem messages?

One of the few positive messages concerns life events. Ever since the late 1960s when Holmes and Rahe[28] presented their work linking life events to subsequent ill-health the topic has aroused much interest. Despite methodological problems,[29] the relationship between life events and subsequent ill-health has been researched in a wide variety of areas ranging from schizophrenia[30] to breast cancer.[31]

Working class women have very high life events rates and also appear particularly vulnerable to the negative effects of life events.[32] Brown and Harris link this with increased rates of depression, but other studies[33] suggest that number of young children in the household, poor relationship with partner at the same time as young children, and lack of paid employment outside the home also contribute to depression, and are also linked with social class. Neither is it possible to separate life events from underlying, long-term difficulties. Loss of home through eviction because of inability to pay rent or make mortgage repayments is usually the climax of long-term financial problems, most frequently contingent upon unemployment. Although unemployment is most usually presented in political and economic terms this denies the underlying moral questions. If unemployment does contribute to ill health, as seems likely, then accepting high unemployment levels for fiscal reasons means adopting a utilitarian approach to health. That many may prosper, and thus be healthy, some must suffer. In some cases, where life events can be predicted, 'anticipatory guidance' can be provided, for example, during pregnancy,[34] or divorce, before retirement or redundancy, or after the event, as in bereavement counselling.[35] For such life events counselling is appropriate and reduces negative outcomes. Where the antecedents are social in origin it would merely be passing the implied 'blame' to the individual.

Work by Brown and his colleagues[32] and others[36] has highlighted the importance of social support as a 'preventive' factor in depression. While it might be ethically dubious to suggest that people should develop their social networks simply to ward off psychological distress, it is unlikely that anyone trying to do so for no other reason would be very successful. Valuing individuals for their unique personal qualities would seem to be inherent in developing relationships. The ability to develop support networks depends not only on the individual's personal qualities, but also on social factors. Living in high-rise flats as well as having young children contribute substantially to isolation, and both are found more in working class women.

On the other hand, the use of self-help groups and support agencies is a growing trend (as discussed by Tountas in Chapter 10), and their use either in time of crisis or to maintain support, and offer information and advice during long-term problems can be invaluable.

From looking at lifestyle characteristics which might minimize distress an obvious step is to move towards targeting mental health messages to subgroups of the population.

TARGETING FOR MENTAL HEALTH EDUCATION

Targeting groups is a well-established technique in health education. In smoking, for example, the target group is children at the age at which they start smoking.[37] What comparable groups might there be in mental health education, and what ethical implications does targeting them have?

Brown's well-known work mentioned above[32] gives some clues and working class women with young children and a poor relationship with their partner are picked out as a vulnerable group. Another at-risk group for depression are those women who have lost their mother during childhood. Can such women be targeted? The cause of vulnerability, the mother's death, cannot be prevented: can its impact be minimized? Apart from telling such women they are vulnerable, what are the clear positive messages?

A further problem in targeting groups is whether the individuals concerned apply the messages to themselves. The stigma involved in admitting to psychological problems or seeking help is probably the first hurdle health educators have to overcome. 'It won't happen to me', 'we've never had anything like *that* in our family' '(psychological problems) only happen to weak characters' are beliefs which mitigate against reaching target populations.

Does pointing out to people they are vulnerable to develop emotional problems encourage the development of such problems? It could be argued that those prone to worrying would worry anyway, about something or other, and this may enable them to direct their worrying into more useful channels.

A growth area in research over the last decade has been stress and its psychological and physical impact. Although much has been written, the nature of the direct link between experienced stress and illness remains controversial. The psychological distress reported, however, is evident. 'The stressed' would thus appear a clear target group. Approaches to managing stress cover a very wide range of options.[38] Leaving these aside for the moment and turning to the causes of stress it is clear that social and occupational roles and pressures contribute to high stress levels in many people.[39] One approach is to help a person accept sources of stress which cannot be changed. The question for those in stress management then becomes not just how to enable a stressed person to cope, but whether a system which contributes to the stress should be bolstered by applying what, in many cases, is the equivalent of a psychological sticking plaster, or whether to work actively to change the system, or to encourage others so to do. The consequences of speaking out must be weighed against possible long-term benefits. In practical terms, for many people, the issue comes down to 'is it worth risking my job, or promotion, to challenge the sources of stress'? This is a value judgment which can only be resolved on an individual basis—both for the stressed person and the health educator. This is not always just a choice between utilitarianism and the good of the individual, but the profit margin (which only directly benefits a minority) versus the health of the workers. The direct and indirect benefits of different economic and political systems are called into question and answers do not always include ethical considerations.

The social factors contributing to mental ill-health are a difficult area for mental health educators and can only be approached at a macro-policy level. By looking at the political environment surrounding the problem, by targeting groups such as the unemployed there is a danger of only treating the symptoms and not causes. If unemployment is deemed to be 'a bad thing' in and of itself, then this will colour approaches to dealing with the problem. An individual's 'right to work' is a political slogan rather than a health one, but it will influence health educators about unemployment and its impact.

Psychiatrists during their training are taught not to fall into the trap of labelling the distress caused by unemployment, poor housing, poverty, and other social problems illness. Limiting distress might be advantageous to the individual, but the distress itself is a reasonable and rational response to social conditions. While psychiatrists might claim that it is not their role to seek to redress social inequalities, a macropolitical stance must be taken by someone. Is this a role for mental health educators?

One group which has been overwhelmingly picked out in mental health programmes has been women. This is not entirely because women present with more psychiatric disorders than men. Our culture allows women to express distress in psychological terms more easily than it allows men, who are more likely to misuse alcohol or show antisocial behaviour,[1] or show stress in somatic form. Women are more likely to use self-help and support groups, thus the situation becomes circular as more groups are provided for those most likely to use them. Some interventions become specifically aimed at women. Assertiveness training is possibly the best example when this is presented as therapy alongside 'behaviour therapy for phobics' and the like in the same journal. It becomes all too easy to link 'being a woman' as 'having a problem' in the same way that 'being phobic' is a problem.

Assertiveness training for women has taken two differing paths. One has adopted a male role model, suggesting that women have to learn male behaviours and attitudes if they are to get on.[40] This model can further undermine women by presenting women and their behaviour as second class. Another approach is more broadly feminist, emphasizing a woman's right to be herself, and usually advocating cooperative behaviours and emotional openness.[41] Two very different ideological standpoints on the same problem. Promotion of either view must surely put forward advantages and disadvantages of both.

It has taken many years for there to be an acknowledgement that many men also lack confidence and want to develop assertiveness skills. This is slowly being responded to.[42]

Possibly because it seems safer ground, most mental health education is targeted at managing illnesses, or clearly defined clinical states. It is also a view which predominates in prevention. Newton,[43] for example, argues persuasively for a disease model approach to preventing mental illness. The mental illness prevention approach raises ethical issues which overlap with those in mental health education, often highlighting them in an extreme way.

MENTAL ILLNESS

It is not possible to discuss ethical issues and mental illness without returning to Cartesian dualism. The divide between body and mind in relation to mental illness is most forcefully, and popularly, expounded by Thomas Szasz. He argues that the proper concern of medicine is physical illness; that since we cannot point to physical causes in mental problems they are, by definition, not illness, and thus mental illness is a myth.[44]

There is not space in this chapter to enter this debate, and it has been discussed most ably elsewhere.[45] The consequences for health education must, however, be faced, for there are two divergent paths. If health educators choose to follow the 'myth of mental illness' path (frequently and often inappropriately called anti-psychiatry) what they seek to do will be very different from those who accept a medical model of mental illness. The former group are frequently portrayed as more liberal than the latter. They oppose involuntary commitment, labelling a person with a 'diagnosis' and, very often, physical treatments, including ECT and drugs.

Szasz's view is not, however, that 'problem' behaviour (labelled by others as ill) should simply be tolerated, but that it is not the role of medicine to police anti-social behaviour in society. If society does not approve of behaviour then it must take steps, through laws and law enforcement, to control such behaviour. Thus not labelling behaviour as 'illness' is not a 'soft option', allowing the perpetrator 'to get away with murder' (sometimes literally).

This is very different from the existentialist or Laingian approach. Laing's view moved from describing schizophrenia as 'a special strategy that a person invents in order to live in an unlivable situation'[46] and the contemporary nuclear family as a 'pathogenic' institution, to seeing schizophrenia as no longer an intrapersonal disease entity but a form of interpersonal functioning,[47] and finally as a political event.[48] At this point, 'true sanity' is found in the person with schizophrenia as they fight against adjustment to 'our alienated social reality'. Schizophrenia is thus described as a transcendental experience: madness is not breakdown but breakthrough. There is no need for therapy, treatment, or rehabilitation.

One of the dangers of this approach (although not to those who advocate it) is that by breaking away from diagnostic labels and calling everything 'distress', the severity of a person's problem can be minimized as the same word applies to those depressed because of appalling social conditions as it does to the person with florid psychotic symptoms. 'Help' (in whatever form) can be denied to the person who wants to adjust to, and live in, this world if the view held is that when a person is schizophrenic the ego has become 'the servant of the divine, no longer its betrayer.'[48]

The various classifications of mental disorders do not make the situation any easier for the public to understand. The distinctions between neurosis, behavioural problems, personality disorders, and psychosis can appear subtle and of no consequence when faced with a person whose behaviour or motivations they cannot understand or do not like. If, however, a strict definition of mental illness is taken, to mean only the psychosis, then comparatively few people fall into this net compared with labelling all psychological distress mentally ill. This latter approach results in the narrowing of the boundaries of the 'normal' as more people are labelled 'ill'.

Much has been written about the abuses of psychiatric diagnosis, particularly schizophrenia, most notably in reference to its political abuse against dissidents in the Soviet Union,[49] the political use in the West against marginalized groups,[50] and the over-representation of blacks through misunderstanding cultural differences.[16,17]

Whether mental and emotional problems are illnesses or not, giving a person a diagnosis has widespread social implications. Governor Dukakis's rating in the opinion polls during the 1988 United States Presidential election campaign dropped considerably when it was rumoured that he had been treated for depression after the death of his brother. The stigma attached to mental illness can limit a person's opportunities, ranging from the job market to their ability to obtain a visa to visit certain countries.

This negative impact has led some psychiatrists to avoid giving patients diagnoses, believing that some vague label such as 'breakdown' or 'emotional problems' causes less damage. It also denies a patient access to information, education, and in some instances, support and advice, and I have argued against this elsewhere.[51]

Many of the secondary problems those with mental illness or other psychological disturbances face stem not from the illness itself but from society's attitudes to them. If society did not stigmatize the mentally ill they may find it easier to live in the community. It is to this end that some mental health education is aimed.

PUBLIC ATTITUDES

The public's negative attitude to the mentally ill is well documented.[52,53] Most studies report the public as believing that the mentally ill are dangerous and unpredictable and people to whom the public do not want to get close. Media descriptions of mental illness tend to emphasize the violence, both in news reporting and documentaries. Although there is some fiction which gives a good account of what it is like to be mentally ill, the emphasis is often on violence or sensationalism. Anthony Perkins in *Psycho* is surely a more enduring image of mental illness than information given by health education agencies.

The reasons why the public have this negative attitude are outwith the scope of this chapter, but the attempts to change these attitudes are not. Most of this is via information aimed at managing particular mental illnesses (or neuroses), for example, schizophrenia, depression, phobia, and anorexia nervosa.[54] Pressure groups, most notably MIND, put forward a view which often refutes the labels of mental illness, preferring such terms as mental distress,[55] and promoting patients' rights, including the right to refuse treatment. Some groups have made television programmes, putting forward such messages as 'We're not mad, we're angry.'[56]

Another view of mental illness is presented by relatives, through organizations such as the National Schizophrenia Fellowship. Many of the relatives speaking through such organizations have severely ill patients with intractable conditions. Their emphasis is on the problems caring for such people brings, and the lack of care and consideration in society.[57,58]

The misunderstanding that the public has over illnesses like schizophrenia, and their antipathy towards it has led a number of relatives to suggest that it would help to change the name. Bleuler's syndrome would, they believe, start life with a clean slate, free from prejudice. Is this really the case?

In the 1970s there was a move to change the name of mongolism to Down's syndrome. That has been a successful relabelling with some apparent change in public attitude. Contributing to this was the racist element of the previous label and new approaches to rehabilitation and education with the mentally handicapped which showed that many could attain skills not previously believed. Over the last few years, however, there has been a move for yet another change of label. People who were previously called mentally handicapped (including those with Down's syndrome) now prefer the label 'people with learning difficulties'.

This raises two points. Firstly, it seems that names have to keep changing to stay ahead of public prejudice. At the end of the day what matters to the public most is not whether someone has schizophrenia or Bleuler's syndrome, is mentally handicapped or has learning difficulties, but whether they behave in what is considered a 'normal', acceptable, or understandable way or not. Whatever the problem is labelled, someone who publicly talks to voices will not be deemed normal.

The second point raised by the change of labelling concerns levels of problems. It is the individual's right to fight prejudice and to describe themselves in terms acceptable to them, and this includes the way society refers to them. If those people who, in archaic terminology would have been labelled 'high grade mental defective' want to be called the manifestly more acceptable 'people with learning difficulties' that is their right. For the most severely mentally handicapped, however, this can appear to be diminishing their problems. For some people, 'learning difficulty' means they can do nothing for themselves, cannot talk, cannot understand what is said to them, cannot feed themselves, are incontinent. To call all people with mental handicap 'people with learning difficulties' is as misleading as to label all people with psychological problems mentally ill, or the mentally ill simply distressed.

Nevertheless, the principle that the public need educating about mental illness with the aim of changing its attitudes and behaviour is an important one. This is an interesting development in health education since it moves away from the utilitarian approach; health education promoting the greatest good for the greatest number. If this is not the principle driving many programmes it is certainly how many campaigns are measured. Targeting at risk groups moves away from the utilitarianism, but in attempting to change the public's attitude to the mentally ill moves further still. Other attitude change campaigns have usually been aimed at putting forward a prevention message to a group which will benefit, ranging from nutrition to seat belts. Other attempts to educate about illnesses (and make them less 'scary') such as cancer, heart disease, and AIDS have also been aimed at those at risk, with the object of individuals taking preventive measures, going for screening, seeking early treatment, and so forth.

The mental illness campaigns have no such positive outcome for those being persuaded to change their attitude (or only very indirectly). The aim is to improve the quality of life of a stigmatized, marginalized group within our society by making that society more tolerant of abnormal behaviour, less frightened of mental problems, more accepting of those who are 'different', and defining what is 'normal' more widely. It may be agreed that by so doing individuals will be able to face their own psychological problems more easily and honestly and that society will be, in some undefined way, 'better'. But to assert this is more a matter of faith than fact.

The issue of the public's attitude to the mentally ill becomes daily more pertinent as the move away from care in institutions to care in the community becomes a reality. Shutting people away in institutions diminishes both the people so isolated and the society which rejects them. Putting people who have been labelled 'different' back into a society ill prepared for them, with not enough resources to provide adequate, let alone good, care, bodes ill for both groups. Society will continue to reject what it does not understand, or does not like (the 'not in my back yard' [NIMBY] syndrome) and the rejected will be left fighting for survival. Breaking this circle of rejection is clearly difficult, but it is the avowed end for many pressure groups and mental health educators.

The move to community care introduces yet another target group for mental health educators, namely the relatives who care for the mentally ill.

CARERS OF THE MENTALLY ILL

Many families are now expected to care for their mentally ill relatives, often with little support from statutory services. There is an increasing volume of research testifying to the burden carried by relatives, not least of which is the effect caring for someone who is mentally ill has on their physical and mental health.[57-59] Problems such as depression, anxiety, guilt, and fear for the future are commonplace. Providing such families with support services can thus be seen as a preventive service, enabling relatives to maintain their own physical and mental health.

The problems of carers are largely tackled by voluntary organizations and charities, although the statutory bodies are gradually accepting the need to provide education and support. The view that people should be cared for by their families and that families should be helped to do this is enshrined in the Griffiths report.[60] One of the many ethical issues embedded in care in the community is that it has been seen by many as essentially 'women's work' and thus promotes the sex-role stereotype of women at home, able to be carers, and not having work outside the home which would interfere with providing this service.[61] The first national survey of carers in Britain however, indicated that a substantial number of men are carers[62] but also showed that male carers have greater access to support services.

It can be difficult for health personnel to offer services to families. Their first responsibility is to the patient, and this includes confidentiality. If a patient denies health personnel access to their family can a service legitimately be offered? One way around this is for information, advice, and support to be offered through another agency, such as health education, so that families can obtain information without compromising doctor-patient relationships. The impact of such support is clearly directed towards relative's understanding and problems, not those of the patients.

CONCLUSIONS

One conclusion which cannot be avoided in this analysis is that ethical issues are integral to every aspect of mental health education. The basic reason for this is that mental health must involve conceptions of the normal and the odd which are not neutral ideas but commit us to value judgments. In other words, the difficulty in defining mental health is not just the difficulty in defining a complex idea but is the ethical difficulty of deciding which aspects of behaviour, emotion, or attitude ought to be promoted and which discouraged.

Does the fact that mental health is difficult to define mean that it should not form part of health education? Even if this view has not been accepted as a matter of principle then a look at current research and programmes seems to indicate that for practical purposes it has been accepted. Many of the causes of distress are rooted in the ethical problems of social disadvantage, gender, and occupational roles which lay burdens on the individual, and cultural expectations which constrict individual expression. The politics of mental health has meant that it is easier to concentrate on recognized and accepted problems and 'illnesses' rather than challenge social, political, and economic powers who control a system which contributes substantially to distress.

An emphasis on individual problems and illness, and individual management of distress can implicitly lay the blame on the intrapsychic functioning of the individual. In physical health an emphasis on healthy diet and exercise indicate that physical fitness does not 'just happen' but is something to be achieved. There are almost no messages in mental health education which are comparable in terms of acceptability and common knowledge. The concept of 'free-floating anxiety' is common in psychiatry as a problem to be diminished. Where is the concept of 'free-floating joy' as a state to be enhanced? To deny the importance of such a concept is to make an ethical rather than a technical judgment.

Health education should be actively pursuing positive mental health. In a world rapidly becoming more homogeneous through international trade and ever more sophisticated channels of communication perhaps one of the most important features of such health promotion should be the acknowledgment of cultural differences in the presentation of positive mental health. Rather than contracting the definition of normality, increased access to other cultures should expand our understanding of the 'normal', encouraging tolerance of a variety of acceptable, healthy behaviours and different routes to well-being. It can be argued that this is of ethical importance not only for the individual, but for society as a whole. The desire for homogeneity may, at the very least, lead to a stagnant society, where novelty is labelled abnormal. At worst it can lead to a repressive society where those who are different are ruthlessly eliminated. Recent European history demonstrates the extremes to which people may go in order to rid themselves of 'deviants'. Nazi Germany may be an extreme example, but a lack of tolerance for individual expression demands an answer to the question of what that society does with those who do not conform. The diversity of both the make-up of positive mental health and the ways of achieving it is something that those working in mental health education must grasp if a way forward is to be found. To do otherwise is to deny ethical principles of individual autonomy and freedom of choice. Utilitarianism is not the only approach in mental health education, although to say we should not abandon the health of a subgroup of society is to take a particular ethical stand. In mental health education every choice is one of ethics.

REFERENCES

1. Briscoe, M.E. Men, women and mental health. *Hlth Educ J* 1985; **44**: 151–153.
2. Harding, C.M. Can health education help to dispel the 'menstrual blues'? *Hlth Educ J* 1984; **43**: 62–66.
3. Milne, D. and Covitz, P. A comparative evaluation of anxiety management materials in general practice. *Hlth Educ J* 1988; **47**: 67–69.
4. Cole, C.W. Community mental health – past, present and future. *Hlth Educ J* 1984; **42**: 99–101.
5. Malin, M.A. and Campion, M.G. Education in human relationships; the case for people with mental handicap. *Hlth Educ J* 1985; **44**: 116–119.
6. Kennedy, A. *Positive Mental Health Promotion. Fantasy or Reality?* Greater Glasgow Health Board Health Education Department, 1988.
7. Dyer, A.R. *Ethics and Psychiatry: Toward Professional Definition*. Washington: American Psychiatric Press, 1988.
8. Nichter, J. Idioms of distress: alternatives in the expression of psychological distress: a case study from South India. *Cult Med Psychiatr* 1981; **5**: 379–408.

9. Teitelbaum, J.M. *Lamta: Leadership and Social Organisation of a Tunisian Community*. Unpublished PhD thesis. University of Manchester, 1960.
10. Orbach, S. *Fat is a Feminist Issue*. London: Hamlyn, 1978.
11. Eysenck, H.J. *The Biological Basis of Personality*. London: C.C. Thomas, 1970.
12. O'Neill, N. and O'Neill, G. *Open Marriage*, New York: Evans, 1972.
13. Comfort, A. *The Joy of Sex*, London: Quartet, 1974.
14. Gordon, C. *Beginner's Guide to Group Sex; Who Does What to Whom and How*. New York: Simon and Schuster, 1974.
15. Tilby, A. Personality clash. *The Listener* 16 March 1989, 10–11.
16. Rach, P. *Race, Culture and Mental Disorder*. London: Tavistock, 1982.
17. Ferando, S. *Race and Culture in Psychiatry*. London: Croom Helm, 1988.
18. Ellis, A. *Reason and Emotion in Psychotherapy*. Secaucus, NJ: Lyle Stuart, 1962.
19. à Kempis, T. *The Imitation of Christ*. London: Dent, 1960.
20. Vitz, P. *Psychology as Religion, The Cult of Self Worship*. Tring: Lion, 1979.
21. Davies, G. *Stress—The challenge to Christian Caring*. London: Kingsway, 1988.
22. Weatherhead, L. *Prescription for Anxiety*. London: Hodder and Stoughton, 1956.
23. Freud, S. Freud's psychoanalytic procedure. In *The Complete Works of Sigmund Freud*. Standard Edition, Vol 7, Translated and edited by J. Strachey. London: Hogarth, 1957.
24. Research Unit in Health and Behavioural Change. *Changing the Public Health*. Chichester: Wiley, 1989.
25. Karasw, T.B. The specificity versus nonspecificity dilemma: toward identifying therapeutic change agents. *Am J Psychiatr* 1986; **143**: 687–695.
26. Beitman, B.D., Goldfried, M.R. and Norcross, J.C. The movement toward integrating the psychotherapies: An overview. *Am J Psychiatr* 1989; **146**: 138–147.
27. Girling, R. Dying for a drink? *Sunday Times Magazine* 19 February 1989.
28. Holmes, T.H. and Rahe, R.H. The social readjustment rating scale. *J Psychoso Res* 1967; **11**: 213–218.
29. Brown, G.W. Meaning, measurement and stressful life events. In Dohrenwend, B.S. and Dohrenwend, B.R. (eds.). *Stressful Life Events: Their Nature and Effect*. London: John Wiley, 1974.
30. Brown, G.W. and Birley, J.L.T. Crises and life changes and the onset of schizophrenia. *J Hlth Soc Behav* 1968; **9**: 203–214.
31. Cheang, A. and Cooper, C.L. Psychosocial factors in breast cancer. *Stress Med* 1985; **1**: 61–66.
32. Brown, G.W. and Harris, T.O. *Social Origins of Depression: A Study of Psychiatric Disorder in Women*. London: Tavistock, 1978.
33. Tennent, C. and Bebbington, P. The social causation of depression: a scriptiques of Brown and his colleagues. *Psychol Med* 1978; **8**: 1–11.
34. Carpenter, J., Aldrich, C.K. and Bovermand, H. The effectiveness of patient's interviews: a controlled study of emotional support during pregnancy. *Arch Gen Psychiatr* 1969; **19**: 110–112.
35. Raphael, B. Preventive intervention with the recently bereaved. *Arch Gen Psychiatr* 1977; **34**: 1450–1454.
36. Cohen, S. and Syme, S.L. *Social Support and Health*. Orlando, Florida: Academic Press, 1985.
37. Goddard, E. and Ikin, C. *Smoking Among Secondary School Children*. OPCS, London: Her Majesty's Stationery Office, 1987.
38. Atkinson, J.M. *Coping with Stress at Work*. Wellingborough: Thorsons, 1988.
39. Cooper, C.L., Lawson, G. and Price, V. A survey of stress at work. *J Soc Occup Med* 1986; **36**: 71–72.
40. Harragan, B.L. *Games Mother Never Taught You*. New York: Rawson, 1977.

41. Dickson, A. *A Woman in Your Own Right. Assertiveness and You*. London: Quartet, 1982.
42. Cornish, C. Standing up for male assertiveness training. *Sunday Times* 12 February 1989.
43. Newton, J. *Preventing Mental Illness* London: Routledge and Kegan Paul, 1938.
44. Szasz. T.S. *The Myth of Mental Illness* London: Secker and Warburg, 1962.
45. Roth, M. and Kroll, J. *The Reality of Mental Illness*. Cambridge: Cambridge University Press, 1986.
46. Laing, R.D.*The Divided Self: A Study of Sanity, Madness and the Family*. London: Davistock, 1960.
47. Laing, R.D. *The Self and Others*. London: Tavistock, 1961.
48. Laing, R.D. *The Politics of Experience*. Harmondsworth: Penguin, 1967.
49. Bloch, S. and Reddaway, P. *Soviet Psychiatric Abuse. The Shadow over World Psychiatry*. London: Gollancz, 1984.
50. Hill, D. *The Politics of Schizophrenia*. Lanham: University Press of America, 1988.
51. Atkinson, J.M. To tell or not to tell the diagnosis of schizophrenia. *J Med Ethics* 1989; **15**: 21–24.
52. Crocetti, G.M., Spiro, H.R. and Siassi, I. *Contemporary Attitudes Toward Mental Illness*. Pittsburgh: Pittsburgh University Press, 1971.
53. Nunnally, J.C., Jr. *Popular Conceptions of Mental Health: Their Development and Change*. New York: Holt, Rinehart and Winston, 1961.
54. Scottish Health Education Group. *Talking About Agrophobia, Talking About Anorexia Nervosa, Talking About Dementia, Talking About Depression, Talking About Schizophrenia*. Edinburgh: SHEG.
55. Byline: Whose Mind is it Anyway? *BBC1*, 1 August 1988.
56. We're Not Mad, We're Angry! *Channel 4*, 17 November 1986.
57. National Schizophrenia Fellowship. *Living With Schizophrenia—by the Relatives*. Surbiton: NSF, 1974.
58. Atkinson, J.M. *Schizophrenia at Home. A Guide to Helping the Family*. London: Croom Helm, 1986.
59. Hicks, C. *Who Cares: Looking After People at Home*. London: Virago, 1988.
60. Griffiths, Sir Roy. *Community Care—Agenda for Action*.—A report to the Secretary of State for Social Services. London: Her Majesty's Stationery Office, 1988.
61. Finch, J. and Groves, D. *A Labour of Love. Women, Work and Caring*, London: Routledge and Kegan Paul, 1983.
62. Green, H. *Informal Carers*. (General Household Survey 1988 GHS No 15 Supplement A). London: Her Majesty's Stationery Office, 1988.

Epilogue

R. S. DOWNIE

Various themes have emerged from the preceding chapters. One concerns the nature of health education itself, which has been shown to involve an understanding of the body, of human growth and development, and of the mind and human behaviour. A second theme concerns the settings for health education: in the home, in schools, in doctors' surgeries, in newspapers and on television, and by government organized campaigns. A third theme, and this one is central to our book, is that ethical considerations are integral to all areas of health education. In her chapter on mental health education Atkinson writes:

'In mental health education every choice is an ethical choice.' (p. 206)

It is hardly an exaggeration to say that one conclusion which has come clearly out of the preceding chapters is that this is true not just of mental health but of all areas in health education.

There are really two aspects to the ethical theme. One concerns the problems which health education by its very nature creates for ethics. Health education is essentially directed at lifestyle and therefore requires to be rendered consistent with our natures as autonomous individuals. Fraudulent claims, dubious expertise, and vested interests whether of governments, commerce, or medicine (orthodox or alternative) can all create a bogus knowledge base which threatens autonomy. High-pressure salesmanship of health can also threaten autonomy. Many of the chapters have been concerned with the various settings for health education in which this problem must be addressed.

The second aspect of the ethical theme concerns the challenges which ethics creates for health education. If our most fundamental ethical value is that of autonomy then this is not something which everyone possesses. Many people are trapped in poor social circumstances and with poor general education. They must be enabled or empowered so that they can develop the ability to make autonomous choices. Health education is one important factor in this process of empowerment. Such a process involves not only the attempt to inform individuals on the workings of their bodies, health service provision, health policies, and environmental factors affecting their health, but also the attempt to combat the powerful anti-health forces in any society. This means that there must be a political dimension to health education. In other words, granted that the enterprise of ethics involves not simply the articulation of static principles safeguarding our autonomy but also the search for dynamic ways in which we can enhance and express our autonomy, then ethics can set the agenda for health education. This is especially so if we remember that health education is concerned not simply with negative health (although that is very important) but with positive health or well-being.

Looking now to the future we can say with confidence that health education is likely to become an increasingly important area of concern over the next decade. This concern is being encouraged firstly by governments and the European Economic Community who have been seen in health education ways of cutting costs. Our own view is that health education is worthwhile regardless of its impact on costs, for health is a value in its own right.

Secondly, the concern is influenced by a distrust of technological medicine and the paternalism which traditionally has gone along with it. The general public increasingly wish to take control of their own lives and health, and are being educated on this by the media—television, radio, newspapers and magazines. Thirdly, other movements, especially environmental ones such as 'Greenpeace' or 'Friends of the Earth' have raised the general consciousness on health matters and the importance of the environment as a health determinant. Finally, public and governmental fears about the spread of AIDS have encouraged varied campaigns on health-related matters. The result of all these influences has been that health education now has a higher profile than it used to have. The fact that health education is set to grow creates opportunities but also problems—practical and ethical—for health education in the 1990s.

Index

Acquired immune deficiency syndrome,
  see AIDS
ADC (AIDS dementia complex), 167
Advertising
  by legal profession, 48–49
  deceptive, victims of, 58–59
  economic pressures for, 45–47
  regulation, 49, 57–58, 59–60
  use of statistics, 51–57
AIDS (acquired immunodeficiency
    syndrome)
  barriers to health education, 162
  epidemiology, 155–156
  introduction, 155
  public knowledge of, 160–161
  risk reduction, ethical issues, 162–165
  summary, 155
  treatment, 96, 97, 157
  WMA on, 85–86
  see also HIV infection
AIDS dementia complex (ADC), 167
AIDS virus screening programme, false
    positives in, 35
AIDS-related complex (ARC), 157
Alcohol
  consumption
    family influence on, 110
    government action, 39
    scientific basis, 188–189
  government revenue from, 72–73
  industries, 71–72
  media presentation of, 185–186
Alcoholism, 147
Anorexia nervosa, 186, 187
ARC (AIDS-related complex), 157
Assertiveness training, 200

Asthma, 147, 148, 149
Autonomy
  doctors and respect for, 31–32
  and health education, 18
  Kant's theory of, 16–17
  modern approach to, 17
  parental authority and child's, 114–117
  political aspects, 65
  professional, 23–24
  versus paternalism in self-care, 146,
    151–152

Beneficence
  doctors and, 32–34
  political attitudes, 33
Black Report, The (HEC), 70
Blood pressure, opportunistic screening,
    30, 36
Breast examination, 30, 34–35, 148

Carers, of the mentally ill, 204–205
Cervical screening, 30, 38
Cheeses, listeria contamination of soft,
    25
Children
  immunization, 31
  influence of family on, 110–112,
    122–123
  parental authority and autonomy of,
    114–117
  television, 112–113, 120–122, 123
  see also Preschool children

Depression, social factors, 198
Diabetes, 147, 148, 149
Dietary fibre, and bowel cancer, 188

211

Disabled, 147
Disease prevention, cost per unit benefit, 38–39
Doctors, 6, 29–40
  and beneficence, 32–34
  examples of ethical problems, 30–31
  limitations, 36–37
  and media, *see* Medical journalism
  and non-maleficence, 34–36
  and preventive medicine, 82
  and respect for autonomy, 31–32
  traditional role, 82
  and withdrawal of treatment, 33–34
Doe, Baby Jane, 96–97
Drug addiction, HIV and intravenous, 159, 160, 161, 162, 165

Eggs, salmonella in, Currie controversy, 24–25, 75
Elderly, self-care in, 148
Emotion, and mental health, 194, 195

Family, influence on children, 110–112, 122–123
Fitness, 4
Food and Drug Administration (FDA), 25, 95
Food safety, 24–26

Haemophiliacs, 149
Handicapped, 147
Health
  in 'grammatical' terms, 141–142
  ill, 3
  nature of, 19–20
  negative, 3, 4
  positive, 3–4
  reasons for valuing, 139–140
  and social class, 69–70, 141
  and unemployment, 71, 198, 200
  and well-being, 5–6
Health care
  advertising
    economic pressures for, 45–47
    regulation of, 57–58, 59–60
    statistics in, 51–57
    victims of deceptive, 58–59
  costs
    increasing, 46–47
    pressures to reduce, 47
  as a right, 39

Health Divide, The (HEC), 70–71
Health education
  criteria, 8–9
  definition, 18–19
    political factors, 64
  and health promotion, 7–8, 10–11
  and medicine, 6–7
  multidisciplinary approach, 18–19
  and nature of health, 19–20
  presentation, 10
  as profession, 65
Health Education Authority (HEA), 74–75
Health education bodies, political independence, 26
Health Education Council (HEC), 64, 68–75
  Beating Heart Disease, 75–77
  foundation, 68–69
  government funding, 69
  product sponsorship by, 73–74
  The Black Report, 70
  The Health Divide, 70–71
Health education officers, 11–12
Health educators, responsibility to, 64–65
Health information, political factors, 75–77
Health professionals
  moral credibility, 184–185
  personal bias, 184
  relationship with patient, 184–185
Health promotion
  and health education, 7, 10–11
  Williams' warning against, 21–22
Heart disease
  Beating Heart Disease, 75–77
  self-help groups, 147, 148
HIV infection
  in Africa, 158–159
  anonymous epidemiological testing, 169–170
  biology of, 156–158
  health education
    evaluation of, 173
    group targeting, 171–172
    safe sex programmes, 172
    in schools, 173–174
    and TV, 174
  in homosexual community, 159, 161, 164
    health education, 172

interrupting spread of, 159–160
intravenous drugs and, *see* Drug
    addiction
mandatory screening debate, 165–171,
    174
  cost–benefit, 169
  test accuracy, 167–169, 170
patterns of, 156
prevalence, 156
social dimensions, 158–159
and STDs, 159, 161
treatment, mandatory, 171
vaccination, 157–158
see also AIDS
Human immunodeficiency virus, *see* HIV
Hypertension, 95, 186

Ill-health, 3
  and social class, 69–70, 141
  and unemployment, 71, 198, 200
Immunization, 31
Individual rights, public welfare versus,
    39–40
Indoctrination
  and health education, 22–23
  nature of, 21–22
International organizations, 87–88, *see
    also* World Medical Association
Ischaemic disease, N-3 polyunsaturated
    fatty acids and, 187–188

Justice, 37–40

Learning, developmental milestones,
    108–109
Life events, and mental health, 198
Lifeskills, 4
Lifestyle
  doctor's influence on, 30, 31
  and media, 185
  and mental health, 194–195, 197
Listeria, in soft cheese, 25

Mammography, 38
Media
  importance in health issues, 93–95
  lifestyle influenced by, 185
  see also Medical journalism;
      Television
Medical ethics, 83–84, *see also* Doctors;
    World Medical Association (WMA)

Medical institutions, and media, 99–101
Medical journalism, 94–103
  AIDS, 96, 97
  changed emphasis, 98
  conclusions, 102
  exploitation of, 95–96, 97
    by doctors, 100
    pharmaceutical industry, 95–96
  introduction, 94–95
  medical institutions and, 99–101
  oversimplification in, 98
  pressures for a 'story', 96
  responsibility in, 95
  summary, 94
  training, 101–102
Medical resources, distribution of, 38
Medicine
  compared to health education, 6–7
  organized
    introduction, 81–82
    summary, 81
    see also World Medical Association
Mental health, 4
  concept, 192–196
  conclusions, 205–206
  development of self and, 193–194
  emotion and, 194, 195
  ethical dilemmas, 196
  individual vs group approach, 196–197
  life events and, 198
  lifestyle and, 194–195, 197
  personality and, 192–193
  politics of, 197–198, 205
  psychotherapy and, 195–197
  religions and, 195
  self-care, 147, 148, 198
  social factors and, 198, 200
  stress, 199
  summary, 191
  targeting, 199–201
  women and, 198, 199, 200
Mental illness
  aetiological factors, 196
  carers, 204–205
  Cartesian dualism and, 192, 201
  as a 'myth', 201
  pressure groups, 203
  public attitudes to, 202–204
  stigma of, 202
  terminology, 203
  see also Mental health

Mentally handicapped, self-care, 147
Microbiological Food Safety, committee on, 25

Non-maleficence, doctors and, 34–36
Nursery school teachers, influence of, 119–120
Nutrition, 181–190
    complexity of influences, 183–184
    direct and indirect education, 182–183
    family influence on, 110
    lifestyle and, 181–182
    media and, 186
    preschool children, 110, 120
    scientific basis for food claims, 186–189
    summary, 181

Obesity
    scientific basis, 187
    self-help, 147, 148
Oral hygiene, child self-care programmes, 148

Parents
    authority over children, 114–117
    concept of health, 117–118
    concept of safety, 118
    education in child healthcare, 118–119
    influence on children, 110–112, 122–123
Personal hygiene, childhood influences, 112
Personality
    early environmental influences, 108
    mental health and, 192–193
Pharmaceutical industry, use of media, 95–96
Political factors
    conclusion, 77–78
    conflicting interests, 68
    freedom from vs freedom for, 66–67
    government revenue from alcohol and tobacco sales, 72–73
    health education
        aims and means, 66
        definition, 64
        ideology in, 67–68
        as profession, 65
        responsibility, 64–65
        in schools, 136–137

    scope of, 66
    health information, 75–77
    HEC as case study, see Health Education Council
    individual vs community, 65
    introduction, 63–64
    justice and inequality, 66
    summary, 63
Poultry, salmonella in, Currie controversy, 24–25, 75
Pregnancy, 31
Preschool children
    accidents and safety, 112
    alcohol and, 110–111
    and daycare influences, 119–120, 123
    exercise and, 111
    and family influences, 110–112
    genetic make-up, 109
    health professionals, attitude to, 111
    introduction, 107–108
    later attitudes to sex, 112
    learning ability, development of, 108–109
    nutrition, 110, 120
    personal hygiene, 112
    recommendations, 122–123
    smoking and, 111
    summary, 107
    taking medicine and, 111
    unconscious learning, 108
    variety of messages aimed at, 119
Psychology, 189, 195
Psychotherapy, mental health and, 195–197
Public health measures, 39

Religions, and mental health, 195

Salmonella, Currie controversy, 24–25, 75
Schizophrenia, 147, 194, 201, 203
Schools, health education, 125–144
    and age, 129
    cigarette smoking, 129–131
    conclusions, 142–143
    and conflict with home values, 137–138
    egocentricity encouraged by, 138
    encouraging healthy lifestyle, 126–127
    HIV infection, 173–174
    introduction, 125–126

justification, 138–142
knowledge base, 129–132
methods, 132–137
objections to, 137–138
political aspects, 136–137
and range of needs, 131
and self-esteem, 139
sex, 129
social benefits of, 140–141
summary, 125
targeting, 130–131
to affect family behaviour, 138
valuing health, 138–139
Schools Council Health Education
    Projects, 135
Screening, 30, 31
false positives, 35
harm/benefits, 34–36
multiphasic medical, 35
opportunistic, 30
Selenium, 188
Self, development of, 193–194
Self-care, 145–154
as alternative way of life, 147
assessment, 148
autonomy versus paternalism, 146,
    151–152
conclusions, 152–153
definition, 146–147
distribution of resources, 146, 149–150
effectiveness, 146, 147–148
groups, 10
ideological and political factors,
    150–151
introduction, 145–146
summary, 145
see also Self-help groups
Self-esteem, 4, 139
Self-help groups
effectiveness, 148
mental health, 198
Sex
education, 129, 193–194

parental attitudes to, 112
Social class
and HEC reports, 70–71
and ill-health, 69–70, 141
Social factors, and mental health, 198,
    200
Social well-being, 4–5
Sociology, 189
Statistics, in healthcare advertising,
    51–57
Stress, 199

Television, and children, 112–113,
    120–122, 123
Tobacco, 19, 30, 32
doctors' use of, 85
education in schools, 129–131
government and, 39, 72–73
industries, 71–72
smoking in nursery schools, 119–120
WMA on, 85, 88–89
Trace elements, 188

Unemployment
and ill health, 71, 198, 200
and social class, 69–70, 141

Well-being, 4–6
social, 5
World Medical Association (WMA),
    84–86
on AIDS, 85–86
Code of Ethics (Helsinki Declaration),
    84–85
Declaration of Geneva, 83, 84–85, 90
on environmental and demographic
    issues, 85, 89–90
International Code of Medical Ethics,
    84, 90–91
and other organizations, 86–87
on tobacco, 85, 88–89
see also Medicine, organized